THE HEALTHY
LIVER&
BOWEL
BOOK

International Edition

Dr Sandra Cabot M.D.

The suggestions, ideas and treatments described in this book are not intended to replace the care and supervision of a trained health care professional. All problems and concerns regarding your health require medical supervision. If you have any pre-existing medical disorders you must consult your doctor before following any suggestions or treatments in this book. If you are taking prescribed medications you should check with your own doctor before using any treatments discussed in this book.

First Published 1999 by
SCB International Inc.: PMB 101 Suite 2A, 13910 North Frank Lloyd Wright Blvd. Scottsdale, Arizona, USA, 85260
Ph: 602 860 4299, 602 770 7246   Website: www.liverdoctor.com

Edition 3 (7/99)

Cartoons by Karen Barboutis

All recipes designed by Audrey Tea are characterised by this symbol ❤

ISBN 0-9673983-0-4

Dedication

This book is dedicated to furthering the understanding and prevention of liver disease.

**The Healthy Liver & Bowel Book
by Dr Sandra Cabot M.D.**

Contents

Section One - The Liver

Chapter One - The Liver and Detoxification ...12

Chapter Two - Liver Dysfunction ...17

Chapter Three - How to Have a Healthy Liver
The Vital Principles for a Healthy Liver ...20
Liver Tonics ...29
The Liver and Weight Loss ...36

Chapter Four - Go Shopping ...39

Chapter Five - Questions and Answers
Gall Bladder Disease ...43
The Gall Bladder Flush ...43
Herbal Teas for the Liver ...47
Livatone and Livatone Plus - The Difference ...48
Boost your Immune System Naturally ...50
Hormone Replacement Therapy and the Liver ...52
Oils and the Liver ...54
Beverages and the Liver ...57
Dining Out ...58
Eggs and Coconut ...59
Calcium Rich Foods ...61
Children and The Liver Cleansing Diet ...63
Liver Cysts ...64
Gilbert's Syndrome ...65
Case Histories ...66
Your Pet's Liver ...68

Chapter Six - Liver Diseases
Liver Tumours ...72
Liver Cancer ...72
Cirrhosis ...73
Hepatitis ...77
How to Prevent Viruses from Damaging your Liver ...82
Haemochromatosis ...84
Wilson's Disease ...87
Sclerosing Cholangitis ...87
Primary Biliary Cirrhosis ...88

Chapter Seven - Metabolism and Cellulite
Metabolic Rate ...90
Factors that Increase Cellulite ...91
Body Type and Cellulite ...93
Natural Supplements to Help Metabolism ...95
Appendix Section One
Liver Function Tests ...99
Liver Help Resources ...100

Section Two - The Bowels

Chapter One - How to have a Healthy Bowel
Causes of Bowel Dysfunction 104
Strategies to Help Bowel Disorders 105
Natural Remedies for the Bowel 110
Bowel Parasites - A Case History 111

Chapter Two - Bowel Problems
Constipation 114
Laxatives 114
Megacolon 115
Inflammatory Bowel Disease 117
    Ulcerative Colitis 117
    Crohn's Disease 119
Irritable Bowel Syndrome 121
Dietary Fibre 124
Prolapsed Colon 126
Peptic Ulcer 127
Reflux 130
Coeliac Disease 131
    Gluten Free Diet 132
Haemorrhoids 135
Diverticulitis 136
Bowel Cancer 138
Bowel Polyps 139
Recovery from Bowel Cancer - A Patients Story 141

Chapter Three - Digestive and Related Problems
Candida 145
High Cholesterol 147
Pancreatitis 150
Diabetes 151
Food Allergies 155

Appendix Section Two:
Tests for Bowel and Digestive Function 158
Colonoscopy/Sigmoidoscopy/Barium Enema/High Salicylate Foods 159

Section Three - The Healthy Liver and Bowel Recipes
Housekeeping with Audrey Tea 164
Beverages - Juices, Smoothies and Teas 168
Breakfasts 174
Soups 181
Dips, Spreads and Dressings 190
Salads, Sides and Snacks 193
Vegetable Mains 212
Poultry 230
Seafood 242
Meat 258
Sweets, Treats and Cakes 263
Appendix Section Three 285
    Measurement Conversion Chart 285
    Organic Food Suppliers/Contact Details 287
Bibliography/References 291
Glossary 295

The Author

Dr Sandra Cabot M.B.B.S., D.R.C.O.G. is a well known media doctor and author of the best-selling books Women's Health, Don't Let Your Hormones Ruin Your Life, The Body Shaping Diet, Menopause - HRT and its Natural Alternatives, Handbag Health Guide, The Liver Cleansing Diet and Boost Your Energy. Her groundbreaking book The Liver Cleansing Diet has sold over one million copies worldwide and won the Australian People's Choice award in 1997. The Liver Cleansing Diet book has been on the Australian best seller list for over two years.

Dr Sandra Cabot is a consultant to the Women's Health Advisory Service, regularly appears on Australian TV shows and with Suzy Yates on radio 2 UE , writes for women's magazines and is a much sought after public speaker on the health issues of our time.

Sandra is sometimes known as the "Flying Doctor" as she frequently flies herself to many country towns to hold health seminars for women and increasingly also for men. These help to raise funds for local community services and women's refuges. Sandra has spent considerable time working in a large missionary hospital in the Himalayan foothills of India.

Sandra receives thousands of letters from people from all over the world who have read her books and are searching for holistic solutions to their health problems.

Her mailing address is PO Box 54 Cobbitty NSW 2570 Australia and her E-mail address is cabot@ozemail.com.au.

Introducing Audrey Tea by Dr Sandra Cabot

The indefatigable Audrey Tea has been cooking delicious and wholesome meals for well over 50 years. Born and bred in Adelaide where Audrey's culinary talents have tantalised the taste buds of thousands, she continues to design and test recipes in collaboration with Dr Sandra Cabot. While maintaining the principles of liver and bowel cleansing nutrition, Audrey can prepare and cook dishes, which range from fabulous family meals, gourmet dinner party menus, quick snacks, special surprises and boutique sweet treats. This skill has taken her many years to perfect yet despite this amazing talent she remains incredibly approachable and giving.

Audrey Tea is also a recipe tester and has had to make many modifications to conventional Western recipes to develop truly liver cleansing and delicious changes to meals that we once used to consider healthy. Audrey helps us to discover that healthy can be gourmet and indeed is usually much tastier and satisfying than the meals that were once considered traditional Australian cuisine. She has managed to make the recipes truly multicultural, which will introduce new flavours and health benefits to you by increasing diversification of your diet.

I have been fortunate to be a recipient of many of Audrey's meals over the years and I hope to continue to receive her regular gifts of treats. I am now delighted to be able to share these recipes with you and your family. They come with laughter and maternal healing vibrations, just like Audrey Tea herself. If you would like to ask Audrey Tea questions about the recipes she has included in this book, identified with a heart ♥, you can write to:

Audrey Tea P. O. Box 54 Cobbitty NSW Australia 2570

Preface

The Healthy Liver and Bowel Book brings you an easy and effective way of eating to live safely in an increasingly toxic world.

How is your body coping at the present moment?

1. Do you feel healthy and energetic all the time?
2. Do you feel unwell and tired all the time?
3. Do you feel below par for more than 50% of the time, and think that you should feel better than you do?

The majority of people answer yes, to the third question, and yet conventional medicine cannot find anything wrong to explain the malaise that currently afflicts millions of people on the planet.

For these people optimum health is like a jig-saw puzzle with a part missing.

Dr. Sandra Cabot M.D. has found after more than 20 years of clinical medicine that the missing part to the jig-saw puzzle of good health is simple and yet often overlooked. She tells us that this missing part is the most strategic organ in the body, and is an organ we have all heard about but do not give the consideration it deserves. This organ is called The Liver and it has everything to do with how well you will live and how long you will live.

To live safely in a toxic world and to avoid the epidemic of immune dysfunction and cardiovascular disease that is affecting millions, you must have a healthy liver to protect you. This book shows you how easy it is to have a healthy liver and digestive system, which will restore good health and fight excessive weight.

Introduction

Many of you will know me from my previous book, titled **The Liver Cleansing Diet** which literally shot to fame like a shining meteorite during 1997. It made me a household name in everyone's kitchen, and brought liver consciousness to hundreds of thousands of people in a short space of time. People from all walks of life and in many different states of health embraced this new and simple way of eating with a passion, that surprised me as well as many others. There are thousands of diet books on the market and yet this one was different because it concentrated on just one bodily organ, namely the liver, which everyone seemed to relate to, because everyone had a liver. Perhaps its success related to the fact that when one improves the liver function through simple dietary habits it is possible to achieve many health benefits, especially weight control and internal cleansing of the body. It was incredible because everyone seemed to be having a love affair with his or her liver. People who had struggled for years with excessive weight and/or chronic health problems found that the liver was the missing part in the jig-saw puzzle to achieve good health.

From that point, word of mouth took over and successful followers of my liver friendly way of eating told others to follow the liver cleansing diet and watched with interest to see its results. This produced a wave of social and economic effects. Australia sold out of linseed (flaxseed) and for a while it had to be imported, health food stores had to knock down walls to create more space and the health food industry enjoyed a resurgence in the production and sales of liver cleansing foods.

I became known as the "liver doctor" which was interesting as my background had been in the area of women's health and hormone replacement therapy. My face became well known, so much so that I would find myself recognised in far-away and remote places. I well remember being in a public toilet at 5am in the morning, at a place called Three Ways, on the highway between Alice Springs and Darwin where I was instantly and warmly welcomed by a woman who had been successful on my liver cleansing diet. She enthusiastically told me how much weight she had lost and how much she enjoyed my media appearances. Yes, one of the benefits of being a successful author is that one has a ready-made network of friends all over the world. On another occasion I was en-route to give a seminar in Newcastle when I had to pop into an RSL club to do a radio interview. It was around 11am and the receptionist kindly let me use the phone, on the condition that I gave her club a plug on the radio. She said to me, "Hi, Doctor Cabot, by the way I have read some of your liver book, and I know that I need it. But can you write something very simple and easy for us really lazy ones, who want to feel and look great without having to think too hard?" So after leaving her club, I thought about this and I decided that this was a good idea. Not everyone wants to do the 8-week plan in my Liver Cleansing Diet book and they may not be interested in all that liver physiology.

I am writing this book on the liver and bowels because it is simple and easy to follow; it will give you the vital principles for a healthy liver and digestive system and a banquet of delicious liver healthy recipes with an infinite amount of variety. You can choose whatever suits your fancy from our huge list of recipes so that you will never have to feel bored or hungry. You can use these recipes for the whole family and they are well balanced and contain all the essential nutrients for a balanced diet. If you have a husband or children who desire foods that are not included in these recipes, you can add those foods as adjuncts to the basic recipes found in this book. For example your husband may enjoy the occasional slice of bacon, piece of pork crackling, or lump of cheese, without which he cannot live, and to keep the peace you may feel obliged to provide these things. Simply add them as a sidepiece to one of our recipes, and he will be more accepting of gradually changing his diet to the liver cleansing way. The same applies to children. Remember that Rome was not built in a day, and it takes time to change one's old habits. The recipes in this book are suitable for children and breast-feeding or pregnant women, and can also be used in those with mature-onset non-insulin dependent (Type II) diabetes.

Those with diabetes and/or severe kidney or liver disease have special nutritional requirements that must be supervised by a dietitian. Women who are pregnant or breast-feeding need to take supplements of iron, calcium and folic acid no matter what diet they are following.

I have collaborated with a brilliant cook by the name of "Audrea Tea", whose culinary talents combined with my "liver know-how", has resulted in the largest collection of addictively yummy recipes to keep both your pleasure centre and mind happy. This is important because if the pleasure centre situated in your brain is not happy with these recipes, you know as well as I do that you will not be able to look after your liver and digestive system for the rest of your life. Your liver is worthy of lots of TLC everyday and indeed being the most important organ in the body we must not neglect it.

Some people do not believe that **The Liver Cleansing Diet** can really work for them, and they read parts of the book, but never try it. Perhaps this is because they do not want to do an 8-week plan, or think that it will be too hard. In reality it is not hard at all; simply follow the vital principles on *page 20 to 27* and use the recipes as guidelines for how you need to cook and eat. You will find it so easy that you will be amazed!

Now if you are suffering with poor health, digestive diseases or a liver problem, you will need to follow this way of eating very accurately for six months to prove to yourself that it works. Put this diet on trial and see for yourself. If it works you will feel and look so much better that you will be delighted, and you will not want to go back to the way you used to be. This eating plan will become a way of life and a way of being in the optimal healthy and non-toxic state, without having to miss out on life's pleasures or subject yourself to excessive discipline.

There has been the occasional person who did not understand my theories on the liver, and in particular one reader thought it was impossible to cleanse the liver, believing that this was unscientific! However, it is vitally important to cleanse the liver regularly because, like any filter, it can become overloaded and blocked with excessive waste products. Just think about what happens if you do not cleanse the filters in your kitchen sink, lawn mower, pool-pump or car engine. It would be easy if you could remove your liver everyday and give it a good wash with soap and water! This is obviously not possible, so we need to come up with a more practical solution.

I have found that an effective way to cleanse the liver filter is by eating certain foods and using natural supplements and liver tonics. By eating the types of foods found in the shopping list and recipes in this book, we are providing the liver with specific nutrients that will help to keep the liver filter healthy, and support the detoxification pathways found inside the liver cells.

These nutrients include anti-oxidants, essential fatty acids, essential amino acids, enzymes, natural antibiotics and plant substances (phytonutrients). These nutrients also exert an anti-cancer effect and help the immune system.

Section One - The Liver

Chapter One - The Liver and Detoxification   ...12

Chapter Two - Liver Dysfunction   ...17

Chapter Three - How to Have a Healthy Liver
    The Vital Principles for a Healthy Liver   ...20
    Liver Tonics   ...29
    The Liver and Weight Loss   ...36

Chapter Four - Go Shopping   ...39

Chapter Five - Questions and Answers
    Gall Bladder Disease   ...43
    The Gall Bladder Flush   ...43
    Herbal Teas for the Liver   ...47
    Livatone and Livatone Plus - The Difference   ...48
    Boost your Immune System Naturally   ...50
    Hormone Replacement Therapy and the Liver   ...52
    Oils and the Liver   ...54
    Beverages and the Liver   ...57
    Dining Out   ...58
    Eggs and Coconut   ...59
    Calcium Rich Foods   ...61
    Children and The Liver Cleansing Diet   ...63
    Liver Cysts   ...64
    Gilbert's Syndrome   ...65
    Case Histories   ...66
    Your Pet's Liver   ...68

Chapter Six - Liver Diseases
    Liver Tumours   ...72
    Liver Cancer   ...72
    Cirrhosis   ...73
    Hepatitis   ...77
    How to Prevent Viruses from Damaging your Liver   ...82
    Haemochromatosis   ...84
    Wilson's Disease   ...87
    Sclerosing Cholangitis   ...87
    Primary Biliary Cirrhosis   ...88

Chapter Seven - Metabolism and Cellulite
    Metabolic Rate   ...90
    Factors that Increase Cellulite   ...91
    Body Type and Cellulite   ...93
    Natural Supplements to Help Metabolism   ...95

Appendix Section One
    Liver Function Tests   ...99
    Liver Help Resources   ...100

Chapter One - The Liver and Detoxification

More than ever before in the history of mankind, human beings need to have healthy livers to break down the chemicals that have crept into our environment. I received an E-mail from a reader of my books, who was alarmed by the large number of hormone implants being inserted into beef animals where she worked in a stock and station agency. Steers are implanted with oestrogens, which is justified by corporate statements, that tests have shown that a non-pregnant woman produces 54,000 times the amount of oestrogen found in a 500 gram steak. This is all very well, however, it is still increasing the workload of the liver, which over a long period of time may cause hormonal imbalances in those who eat beef regularly. We must ask ourselves why is the incidence of breast cancer so high, particularly in relatively young women? Surely it is better to eat meat from animals that roam free and happy in fresh green pastures that are not injected with potent hormones or fed concentrated stock feed to rush their growth?

The liver is the gateway to the body and in this chemical age its detoxification systems are easily overloaded. Thousands of chemicals are added to food and over 700 have been identified in drinking water. Plants are sprayed with toxic chemicals, animals are injected with potent hormones and antibiotics and a significant amount of our food is genetically engineered, processed, refined, frozen and cooked. All this can lead to destruction of delicate vitamins and minerals, which are needed for the detoxification pathways in the liver. The liver must try to cope with every toxic chemical in our environment, as well as damaged fats that are present in processed and fried foods.

The Liver Filter

The liver is the cleanser and filter of the blood stream and is of vital importance.

The liver is the largest organ in the body and has an enormous amount of blood flowing through it every minute of our lives.

If we examine the liver under a microscope, we will see rows of liver cells separated by spaces which act like a filter or sieve, through which the blood stream flows. The liver filter is designed to remove toxic matter such as dead cells, microorganisms, chemicals, drugs and particulate debris from the blood stream. The liver filter is called the sinusoidal system, and contains specialised cells known as Kupffer cells (*see colour diagram between pages 64 and 65*), which ingest and breakdown toxic matter. The liver filter can remove a wide range of microorganisms such as bacteria, fungi, viruses and parasites from the blood stream, which is highly desirable, as we certainly do not want these dangerous things building up in the blood stream and invading the deeper parts of the body. Infections with parasites often come from the contaminated water supplies found in large cities, and indeed other dangerous organisms may find their way into your gut and blood stream from these sources. This can cause chronic infections and poor health, so it is important to protect your liver from overload with these microorganisms. The safest thing to do is boil your water for at least 5 minutes, or drink only bottled water that has been filtered and sterilised. High loads of unhealthy microorganisms can also come from eating foods that are prepared in conditions of poor hygiene by persons who are carrying bacteria, viruses or parasites on their skin. Foods, especially meats that are not fresh or are preserved, also contain a higher bacterial load, which will overwork the liver filter if they are eaten regularly.

Recently, it has become very fashionable for people to detoxify their bodies by various means, such as fasting or cleansing the bowels with fibre mixtures. Fasting can by its extreme nature, only be a temporary method of cleansing the body of waste products, and for many people causes an excessively rapid release of toxins which can cause unpleasant, acute symptoms. The liver filter, like any filter, needs to be cleansed regularly, and it is much easier and safer to do it everyday. This is easily and pleasantly achieved by adopting a daily eating pattern that maintains the liver filter in a healthy clean state. By following the recipes, methods of cooking, and guidelines in this book, you will be able to keep the liver filter healthy and clean. Although it is important to keep the intestines moving regularly and to sweep their walls with high fibre and living foods, it is important to remember that the bowels are really a channel of elimination and not a cleansing organ per se. In other words the bowels cannot cleanse, filter or remove toxic wastes from the blood stream.

It is only the liver that can purify the blood stream and we only have one liver.

The Liver Detoxification Pathways

Inside the liver cells there are sophisticated mechanisms that have evolved over millions of years to break down toxic substances. Every drug, artificial chemical, pesticide and hormone, is broken down (metabolised) by enzyme pathways inside the liver cells.

Many of the toxic chemicals that enter the body are fat-soluble, which means they dissolve only in fatty or oily solutions and not in water. Fat-soluble chemicals have a high affinity for fat tissues and cell membranes, which are made of fatty substances. In these fatty parts of the body, toxins may be stored for years, being released during times of exercise, stress or fasting. During the release of these toxins, symptoms such as headaches, poor memory, stomach pain, nausea, fatigue, dizziness and palpitations may occur.

The liver is designed to convert fat-soluble chemicals into water-soluble chemicals so that they may then be easily excreted from the body

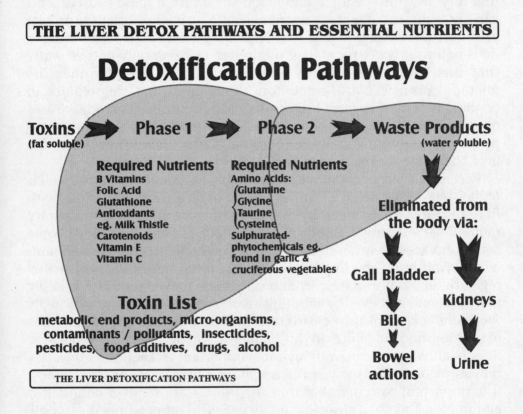

THE LIVER DETOX PATHWAYS AND ESSENTIAL NUTRIENTS

Detoxification Pathways

Toxins (fat soluble) ➤➤ **Phase 1** ➤➤ **Phase 2** ➤➤ **Waste Products** (water soluble)

Required Nutrients
B Vitamins
Folic Acid
Glutathione
Antioxidants
eg. Milk Thistle
Carotenoids
Vitamin E
Vitamin C

Required Nutrients
Amino Acids:
Glutamine
Glycine
Taurine
Cysteine
Sulphurated-phytochemicals eg. found in garlic & cruciferous vegetables

Eliminated from the body via:

Gall Bladder

Kidneys

Bile

Urine

Bowel actions

Toxin List
metabolic end products, micro-organisms, contaminants / pollutants, insecticides, pesticides, food additives, drugs, alcohol

THE LIVER DETOXIFICATION PATHWAYS

via watery fluids such as bile and urine.

How the Liver Detoxifies Harmful Substances

Basically there are TWO major detoxification pathways inside the liver cells, which are called the Phase 1 and Phase 2 detoxification pathways (*see diagram above*).

Phase One - Detoxification Pathways

An example of the phase one pathway is the Cytochrome P-450 mixed function oxidase enzymes. This pathway converts a toxic chemical into a less harmful chemical. This is achieved by various chemical reactions (such as oxidation, reduction and hydrolysis), and during this process free radicals are produced which, if excessive, can damage the liver cells. Antioxidants (such as vitamin C and E and natural carotenoids) reduce the damage caused by these free radicals. If antioxidants are lacking, toxic chemicals become far more dangerous.

Excessive amounts of toxic chemicals such as pesticides can disrupt the P-450 enzyme system.

Phase Two - Detoxification Pathway

This is called the conjugation pathway, whereby the liver cells add another substance (eg. cysteine, glycine or a sulphur molecule) to a toxic chemical or drug, to render it less harmful. This makes the toxin or drug water-soluble, so it can then be excreted from the body via watery fluids such as bile or urine. Through conjugation, the liver is able to turn drugs, hormones and various toxins into excretable substances. For efficient phase two detoxification, the liver cells require sulphur-containing amino acids such as taurine and cysteine. The nutrients glycine, glutamine, choline and inositol are also required for efficient phase two detoxification. Eggs and cruciferous vegetables (eg. broccoli, cabbage, Brussels sprouts, cauliflower), and raw garlic, onions, leeks and shallots are all good sources of natural sulphur compounds to enhance phase two detoxification. Thus, these foods can be considered to have a cleansing action.

The phase two enzyme systems include both UDP-glucuronyl transferase (GT) and glutathione-S-transferase (GSH-T). Glutathione is the most powerful internal antioxidant and liver protector. It can be depleted by large amounts of toxins and/or drugs passing through the liver, as well as starvation or fasting.

Toxic Overload

If the phase one and two detoxification pathways become overloaded, there will be a build up of toxins in the body. Many of these toxins are fat-soluble and incorporate themselves into fatty parts of the body where they may stay for years, if not for a lifetime. The brain and the endocrine (hormonal) glands are fatty organs, and are common sites for fat-soluble toxins to accumulate. This may result in symptoms of brain dysfunction and hormonal imbalances, such as infertility, breast pain, menstrual disturbances, adrenal gland exhaustion and early menopause. Many of these chemicals (eg. pesticides, petrochemicals) are carcinogenic and have been implicated in the rising incidence of many cancers.

If the filtering and/or detoxification systems within the liver are overloaded or inefficient, this will cause toxins, dead cells and microorganisms to build up in the blood stream. This will then increase the workload of the immune system, which will become overloaded and irritated. The immune system will then produce excessive inflammatory chemicals, and in some cases, autoantibodies, because it is in a hyper-stimulated state. This may lead to symptoms of immune dysfunction such as allergies, inflammatory states, swollen glands, recurrent infections, chronic fatigue syndrome, fibromyalgia or autoimmune diseases. Some of the more common autoimmune diseases are systemic lupus erythematosus (SLE), sclerosing cholangitis, primary biliary cirrhosis, Hashimoto's thyroiditis, vasculitis and rheumatoid arthritis.

Immune dysfunction is common in the chemically overloaded environment we live in today, and is exacerbated by nutritional deficiencies inherent in processed and high fat diets. Suppressive drugs are often used to treat symptoms of immune dysfunction.

Rarely does anyone think about the liver,
which seems incredible to me because it is such a
powerful organ and is easily improved. Indeed the simplest
and most effective way to cleanse the blood stream
and thus take the load off the immune system is
by improving liver function.

Chapter Two - Liver Dysfunction

Liver Problems are Common

The liver has everything to do with how we live, that's why it is called the liver. The state of your liver will have a huge bearing upon how well you live, how long you will live and how you will look and feel.

In todays world, the liver has to work harder than ever before, and all over the world we find that liver problems are increasing. Globally, one in every ten persons suffers with some type of liver, bile duct or gall bladder disease. Liver cancer is one of the most common cancers in men and has a poor outlook.

350 million people worldwide suffer from hepatitis B which kills more than 2 million annually. Hepatitis C is the most rapidly spreading infectious disease in many countries and is a time bomb waiting to explode. These problems are increasing, and thousands of people are waiting anxiously for liver transplants that many of them will never be lucky enough to receive. There are just not enough donor livers to keep up with the demand.

Liver Dysfunction

This is different to liver disease in that the liver has not yet sustained permanent or sufficient damage to cause gross impairment of its vital functions. In those with a dysfunctional liver, the routine blood tests of liver function are generally normal.

A dysfunctional liver is not working efficiently, and is overloaded, toxic or sluggish. Liver dysfunction is much more common than liver disease, and may be a forerunner to liver disease. In my experience of over 20 years of clinical medicine, I have found that approximately one in every three persons has a dysfunctional liver. Even if the level of dysfunction is only slight, it will still have a negative impact on your immune system and energy levels.

Many people suffer with the symptoms and signs of a dysfunctional liver for years, and yet the treating doctor or naturopath does not recognise the significance of these symptoms. The result is that the symptoms get treated while the underlying problem of an overloaded, toxic and inefficient liver is ignored or only partially treated. Inevitably, the patient's symptoms deteriorate, and increasing doses of drugs such as antibiotics, anti-inflammatory medication, immune-suppressants, pain killers, cholesterol lowering drugs etc, are needed.

The full range of symptoms indicative of "dysfunctional liver syndrome" can only be defined after a study of Eastern and Western medical disciplines. Chinese doctors have long considered the liver to be the most important organ in the body and indeed they call the liver, the "General of the Army" of the body. I consider the liver to be the most strategic organ in the body, because by improving its function we are able to help many other body systems.

Symptoms associated with Liver Dysfunction

1 Abnormal Metabolism of Fats

Abnormalities in the level of fats in the blood stream, for example, elevated LDL cholesterol and reduced HDL cholesterol and elevated triglycerides.

Arteries blocked with fat, leading to high blood pressure, heart attacks and strokes.

Build up of fat in other body organs (fatty degeneration of organs).

Lumps of fat in the skin (lipomas and other fatty tumours).

Excessive weight gain, which may lead to obesity.

Inability to lose weight even while dieting.

Sluggish metabolism .

Protuberant abdomen (pot belly).

Cellulite.

Fatty liver.

Roll of fat around the upper abdomen - (liver roll).

2 Digestive Problems

Indigestion.

Reflux.

Haemorrhoids.

Gall stones and gall bladder disease.

Intolerance to fatty foods.

Intolerance to alcohol.

Nausea and vomiting attacks.

Abdominal bloating.

Constipation.

Irritable bowel syndrome.

Pain over the liver - (upper right corner of abdomen & lower right rib cage).

liver roll

3 Blood Sugar Problems

Craving for sugar.

Hypoglycaemia and unstable blood sugar levels.

Mature onset diabetes (TypeII) is common in those with a fatty liver.

4 Nervous System

Depression.

Mood changes such as anger and irritability. Metaphysically the liver is known as the "seat of anger".

Poor concentration and "foggy brain".

Overheating of the body, especially the face and torso.

Recurrent headaches (including migraine) associated with nausea.

5 Immune Dysfunction

Allergies - sinus, hay fever, asthma, dermatitis, hives, etc.

Multiple food and chemical sensitivities.

Skin rashes and inflammations.

Increased risk of autoimmune diseases.

Chronic Fatigue Syndrome.

Fibromyalgia.

Increase in recurrent viral, bacterial and parasitic infections.

6 External Signs

Coated tongue.

Bad breath.

Skin rashes.

Itchy skin (pruritus).

Excessive sweating.

Offensive body odour

Dark circles under the eyes.

Yellow discolouration of the eyes.

Red swollen itchy eyes (allergic eyes).

Acne rosacea -

(red pimples around the nose, cheeks and chin).

Brownish spots and blemishes on the skin (liver spots).

Red palms and soles which may also be itchy and inflamed.

Flushed facial appearance or excessive facial blood vessels (capillaries/ veins).

7 Hormonal Imbalance

Intolerance to hormone replacement therapy or the contraceptive pill (eg. side effects).

Menopausal symptoms such as hot flushes may be more severe.

Premenstrual syndrome may be more severe.

NOTE:

All of the above symptoms are common manifestations of a dysfunctional liver. However, they can also be due to other causes, of a more sinister nature, so, in all cases of persistent symptoms it is vital to see your doctor.

The Vital Principles
for a
Healthy Liver

• Think Raw

Eat plentiful amounts of raw fruits and vegetables, especially dark green leafy vegetables and orange, yellow, purple and red coloured fruits and vegetables. Thirty to forty percent of the diet should consist of raw fruits and vegetables. Try to eat some raw fruits or vegetables with EVERY meal as they contain living enzymes, vitamin C, natural antibiotic substances and anti-cancer phytonutrients.

• Oil but Don't Grease Your Body

Avoid the fats that present a high workload for the liver and gall bladder. These are full-cream dairy products, margarines, processed vegetable oils (hydrogenated fats), deep fried foods, foods that are not fresh and contain rancid fats, preserved meats, animal skins and fatty meats. In those with a dysfunctional liver, I recommend avoiding all animal milks and substituting them with oat, rice, almond or soymilks.

Eat the "good fats" which contain essential fatty acids
in their natural unprocessed form.

These are found in cold pressed vegetable and seed oils, avocados, fish (especially oily fish such as salmon, tuna, sardines, herring, sablefish, flounder, trout, bass and mackerel), shrimp, prawns and crayfish, raw fresh nuts, raw fresh seeds such as flaxseeds (linseeds), sunflower seeds, safflower seeds, sesame seeds, hemp seeds, alfalfa seeds, pumpkin seeds and legumes (beans, peas and lentils). Seeds such as flaxseeds can be ground freshly everyday (in a regular coffee grinder or food processor) and can be added to cereals, smoothies, fruit salads and vegetables. Spirulina, evening primrose oil, black currant seed oil, borage oil and lecithin also contain healthy oils to help the liver.

Do not use butter and/or margarine on your breads and crackers. Replace them with tahini, humus, pesto, tomato paste or relish, freshly minced garlic and cold pressed oil (chilli or other natural spices can be added if enjoyed), nut-spreads, fresh avocado, cold pressed olive oil or honey.

The good fats are essential to build healthy cell membranes around the liver cells. As we get older we need to "oil" our bodies and not "grease" our bodies.

• Think Natural

Avoid artificial chemicals and toxins such as insecticides, pesticides, and artificial sweeteners and colourings, (especially aspartame), flavourings and preservatives. Excess alcohol, particularly spirits, should be avoided. There is an excellent book called "Chemical Free Living" by Trixie Whitemore, published by Milner Publishing, which shows you how to avoid chemicals in the home.

• Be Diverse

Consume a diverse range of proteins from grains, raw nuts, seeds, legumes, eggs, seafood, and if desired, free range chicken (without the skin), and lean fresh red meats. If you do not want to eat red meat or poultry this is quite acceptable as there are many other sources of protein.

It is safe to be a strict vegetarian, however you may need to take supplements of vitamin B 12, iron, taurine and carnitine to avoid poor metabolism and fatigue.

To obtain first class protein, strict vegetarians need to combine 3 of the following 4 food classes at one meal - grains, nuts, seeds and legumes, otherwise valuable essential amino acids may be deficient. If your body is lacking amino acids you will be fatigued and you may suffer with mood changes, reduced cognitive function, hypoglycaemia, poor immune and liver function and hair loss. I have met many strict vegans who felt unwell because they were lacking amino acids, iron and vitamin B 12, and after supplementing with these nutrients and modifying their diets they quickly regained excellent health.

• Let Food Be Your Medicine

Many diseases can be overcome by eating healing foods that contain powerful medicinal properties. Optimal health and the prevention of disease is only possible by including these healing foods regularly in the diet. The healing substances found in certain foods or therapeutically active chemicals are known as phytochemicals.

The culinary habits of different cultures have been recognised for decades as being influential in the incidence of diseases. Mediterranean countries have a lower prevalence of cardiovascular diseases because of the protective effect of traditional Mediterranean foods, such as olive oil, tomatoes and legumes. Broccoli and other vegetables in the cruciferous family are known to reduce the risk of bowel cancer, but it is only recently that scientists have isolated the phytochemicals which confer this protection. Broccoli has been found to contain a phytochemical called sulphoraphane, which enhances the phase two-detoxification pathway in the liver. Sulphoraphane has also been found to block mammary tumour formation in rats.

Tomatoes contain a powerful antioxidant called lycopene, which according to a paper published in the American Journal of Clinical Nutrition (1997:66:116-22), is the most powerful of all the dietary carotenoids. The researchers found that the dietary intake of lycopene was linked to a lower risk of prostate problems. They also found that higher levels of lycopene in the blood lowered the risk of cell proliferation, which would theoretically exert a powerful anti-cancer effect. Cooking or chopping tomatoes increases the absorption of lycopene into the body. Cooking tomatoes in oil increases the availability of the lycopene to the body, which is another reason that Mediterranean cuisine confers health benefits.

Beetroot is a beautiful deep purple colour because it contains the antioxidant anthocyanidin. Constituents of beetroot have been shown to exert anti-viral and anti-tumour effects in animal studies. Other foods, which also exert these properties, although to a lesser degree, are red and green peppers, red onion skins, paprika and cranberry. These foods contain healing phytonutrients such as carotenoids, capsanthin and anthocyanins.

Certain foods have high concentrations of plant hormones, which are known as phytoestrogens. Examples of these are the isoflavones genistein and daidzein (found in soya beans and red clover), and lignans (found in flaxseed). Asian communities consume a high intake of soy (approximately 25 - 50 grams daily), and have a significantly lower incidence of hormone-dependent cancers of the prostate, uterus and breast. All legumes such as beans, peas and lentils contain beneficial phytoestrogens.

A study published in the British Medical Journal in 1990, looked at a group of postmenopausal women who were given 45 grams of soy flour for 2 weeks, followed by 25 grams of flaxseed meal for 2 weeks, and then 10 grams of red clover sprouts. This produced improvements in various blood hormone levels and menopausal symptoms.

Asian and Mediterranean cuisines are now integrating themselves into the old fashioned Western diet consisting of meat, bread and 4 vegetables. This culinary multiculturalism has enormous and proven benefits for our health and also for our enjoyment. We all know that variety is the spice of life, and Asian and Mediterranean foods can add spice to our often-bland ways of eating. A wide range of Asian foods is now available from supermarkets and greengrocers as well as Chinese grocery stores. Typical

Asian foods and vegetables such as ginger root, chilli, garlic, Chinese water spinach, bok choy, lemongrass, coconut, tumeric, curry, Chinese mushrooms and many others can be experimented with, and gradually introduced into the diet if you want to expand the horizons of your taste buds.

• Watch That Sweet Tooth

Use natural sugars from fresh fruits and juices, dried fruits, honey, molasses, fruit sorbets, fruit cakes, fruit jams, carob, date sugar, maple sugar or syrup or rice syrup. Avoid refined white sugar and candies, fizzy drinks, cakes and biscuits made with refined sugars.

• Rehydrate Your Body

Drink large amounts of fluids such as water, raw juices and teas (green tea, herbal and regular weak tea is fine). Aim for 2 litres of fluid daily and this will avoid constipation problems and help your kidneys to eliminate the toxins that the liver has broken down. Use a household water filter. Water filters with sub-micron, solid carbon block filters are able to remove parasites and many toxic chemicals. Shop around and take a look at different types of filters before you buy and get professional advice as technology is improving rapidly.

The liver is the major organ involved in detoxification, however it is still important to support the other body organs of elimination. The skin and the kidneys eliminate toxins through sweating and urine and this is why saunas and a high intake of filtered water can reduce symptoms of toxic overload.

• Go Organic

Not many people want to eat fruits and vegetables that have been sprayed repeatedly with insecticides and fungicides, ripened with ethylene gas and perhaps waxed with an insect secretion. It is a little off putting while biting into your lovely red juicy steak to think that this animal may have been fed antibiotics and the ground-up remains of thousands of dead animals, and had potent sex hormones implanted into it to accelerate its growth. The healthy reputation of meat was tarnished by the epidemic of mad cow disease (BSE) that has been troubling England and other parts of Europe for some years now. In 1996, the British government conceded that BSE could possibly pass to humans and cause a fatal type of dementia called Creutzfeldt Jakob Disease (CJD). The British government has banned farmers from feeding livestock the remains of dead cattle, and the use of meat and bone meal as an agricultural fertiliser. Dr. Carleton Gadjusek, noted for his Noble Prize winning research, believes that a form of BSE could manifest in chickens and pigs fed the melted down remains of many animals found in meat and bone meal. The disease may not be obvious because the animals are slaughtered before the disease has time to develop. **Ref 19**. There are differing opinions regarding the causes and transmission of BSE and CJD, as it is difficult to detect in infected animals. For these important reasons it would be prudent to implement a worldwide total ban on feeding any animal tissue to livestock, as the WHO has called for.

Organic food is sometimes called biodynamic food and is produced without synthetic herbicides, insecticides, fertilisers, post-harvest fungicides, antibiotic growth-promoters, or size enhancing hormones. It relies upon Mother Nature's forces, recycling of nutrients and sustainable methods of production. Foods certified as organic must be grown on farms that are inspected and fully certified according to a stringent set of standards. Packaged and/or processed organic foods are free from artificial preservatives, colourings, flavourings or additives, and should not contain irradiated or genetically modified ingredients. For information on organic growers and their certifying bodies *see page 287.*

• Keep Your Bowels Moving

Avoid constipation by having plenty of fibre found in unprocessed food and raw fruits and vegetables. One really good trick to keep your bowels moving is to grind flaxseed (linseed), sunflower seeds and almonds (LSA), in a coffee grinder to produce a fine powder, and eat 2 to 3 tablespoons of this powder daily. You can add other ground up seeds, that are high in fibre such as psyllium, pumpkin, sesame and alfalfa seeds to increase the fibre content of the powder. Add this powder to smoothies, vegetables, soups, cereals and fruit salads. Other good sources of fibre are brans made from wheat, oats, soy or rice. Sweet corn either raw or freshly and lightly cooked, is an excellent source of bowel cleansing fibre. Fibre acts like a broom in your bowels and sweeps their walls clean of accumulated layers of waste products, which can then be eliminated in the bowel actions (faeces).

• Be a Gourmet not a Gourmand

Be selective and aim for food taste and quality, instead of quantity. Chew slowly so that you can tune into the subtle tastes of natural foods, oils, spices and herbs. All of the recipes in this book are delicious, and will tempt you to eat slowly to savour their ingredients.

Do not overeat, and listen to the messages from your body. When you feel full and satisfied stop eating. Consistently overeating greatly increases the workload of the liver, and this may reduce its capacity to detoxify harmful substances efficiently. Overworking the liver also reduces its ability to burn fat so that you will be more likely to develop a "fatty liver". Many people unwittingly "dig their grave with their teeth".

• Pamper Your Liver

Eat foods to increase nutrients beneficial to liver function. These are:

Vitamin K - green leafy vegetables and alfalfa sprouts.

Arginine - this helps the liver to detoxify ammonia, which is a toxic waste product of protein metabolism. Arginine is found in legumes (beans, peas, and lentils), carob, oats, walnuts, wheatgerm and seeds.

Antioxidants - found in fresh raw juices such as carrot, celery, beetroot, dandelion, apple, pear and green drinks like wheatgrass and barley-grass juice, and fresh fruits, particularly citrus and kiwi fruit.

Selenium - sources of the antioxidant selenium are brazil nuts, brewers yeast, designer yeast powders (very good source), kelp, brown rice, molasses, seafood, wheatgerm, whole-grains, garlic and onions.

Methionine - is essential for detoxification. Is found in legumes, eggs, fish, garlic, onions, seeds and meat.

Essential fatty acids - Seafood, cod liver oil, and fish oil. Seafood may be fresh, canned or frozen such as sardines, salmon, mackerel, tuna, trout, mullet, blue mussels, calamari, tailor, herring, blue eye cod, gemfish. Fresh avocado, fresh raw nuts and seeds, legumes (beans, peas, lentils), wholegrain, wheatgerm, green vegetables such as spinach, green peas and green beans, eggplant, cold pressed fresh vegetable and seed oils, freshly ground seeds, especially flaxseeds (linseed), evening primrose oil, black-currant seed oil, star flower oil. Essential fatty acids are required for healthy membranes in every cell of the body and plentiful amounts are required for healthy liver function. This is why strict low fat diets are not beneficial for general health, weight control or liver function.

Natural sulphur compounds - are found in eggs (preferably free range), garlic, onions, leeks, shallots and cruciferous vegetables such as broccoli, cauliflower, cabbage and Brussels sprouts.

• Practice Good Hygiene

The liver filter removes microorganisms from the blood stream, which prevents them from getting deeper into the body where they may cause serious infections. To avoid overloading the liver filter it is important to avoid eating foods that are contaminated with high loads of unfriendly or dangerous (pathogenic) microorganisms.

Although standards of living and sanitation have improved, cases of food poisoning from parasites, bacteria and viruses have been gradually increasing. This is often due to poor hygiene, such as inadequate cleansing of areas where food is prepared and stored, and lack of hand washing before preparing and eating food. This is more common today because people have a false sense of security brought about from antibiotic drugs, however many new viruses and pathogenic bacteria resistant to antibiotics are emerging.

The excessive practise of feeding antibiotics to animals is contributing to the rising incidence of antibiotic resistant strains of bacteria such as E.coli, Staphylococcus and Salmonella. Other microorganisms that can cause food poisoning are Campylobacter, Listeria, Yersinia, Clostridium Botulinum and Shigella. Food poisoning can also occur from the toxins produced by some bacteria, algae and moulds. Shellfish grown in waters polluted with toxic algae bloom can accumulate their toxins, which can cause severe neurological dysfunction. Foods contaminated by certain moulds or fungi, which produce their own mycotoxins, can make you sick. The fungus Aspergillus flavus produces the dangerous mycotoxin called aflotoxin. This can grow on damp maize, wheat, corn, peanuts and some other crops.

People are eating out more and there is less cooking done in the home so it is difficult to control standards of food preparation for your family.

People purchase foods from supermarkets where food may have travelled long distances and be stored or refrigerated for long periods, picking up microorganisms along the way. Many processed foods contain preservatives, which do not eradicate microorganisms, but merely keep them in a dormant state. When this food gets into your intestines the preservatives are diluted and the bugs start to multiply. This is why it is important to purchase only fresh high quality foods.

The risk of food contamination is increased by long storage times, the number of people who handle and package food, and inadequate cooling and re-heating temperatures.

The intensive mass production of animal meats has helped to spread infections in food supplies. Chickens fed stock-feed infected with the bacteria Salmonella (sometimes from the remains of other chickens), allow bacteria to recycle and multiply in the same way that cow cannibalism caused the epidemic of mad cow disease (BSE). Chickens infected with Salmonella or viruses, and other animals reared in crowded conditions, can easily cross-infect each other while alive or at the abattoir. John Pattison, chairman of Britain's BSE Advisory Committee believes that mad cow disease (BSE) spread in England from infected hamburger meat made with every part of an animal.

Tips For Good Hygiene

Wash your hands thoroughly with soap and hot water before preparing and eating food, and after handling any raw meat or seafood. Brushing under the nails with a nailbrush can remove inaccessible bacteria.
Wash kitchen utensils such as cutting boards, grinders, juicers, and blenders and can openers thoroughly after each use. Replace cloths, bottlebrushes, pot scratchers and wettexes used to wash dishes frequently.

• Only purchase fresh foods and avoid foods that are mouldy or look too old. Avoid processed or preserved meats such as hamburger meat, ham, smoked and pickled meats and fish, beef jerky, bacon, sausages, fritz, cabanossi, pizza meats, corned beef, meat loaf, rolled meats as found in delicatessens, and sea food that has been mishandled or poorly stored.
• Do not let food stand in warm temperatures for more than two hours.
• Hot foods should be cooled quickly at room temperature and then refrigerated, because gradual cooling allows microorganisms to grow. For the same reasons, do not eat food that has been cooked, cooled and reheated more than once. It is times like these that pet dogs and cats are great for recycling food.
• Refrigerate raw meat, seafood or chicken as soon as possible to reduce bacterial multiplication.
• Defrost poultry, seafood or meat in a microwave oven or overnight in the refrigerator and not on a counter.
• Cook all poultry, seafood and meat thoroughly because the centre of the food must reach 70°C (158°F) to kill bacteria.
• Store raw meat and poultry at a lower level in the refrigerator to avoid their juices contaminating other foods.
• Always refrigerate eggs and foods containing eggs, and discard eggs with cracks.
• Avoid nuts with mould on their shell or kernel, or those with a bitter taste.
• Boil for 5 minutes all tap water used for drinking, food preparation and cooking.
• Use antiseptics when cleaning the toilet, bath and shower recess. Antiseptic soaps can be used in large households or share type accommodation. Tea tree oil has useful antiseptic properties, and effective antiseptics are easily found in supermarkets and pharmacies at reasonable prices. Avoid sharing toothbrushes and razor blades as serious blood borne infections can be transmitted this way.

Improve your Liver Function

Liver Tonics

These are helpful for the liver in many ways and are best obtained in powder and capsule form. A good liver tonic needs to contain a synergistic mixture of natural ingredients, which work together to support liver function. There are many liver tonics available, from Swedish bitters to tinctures containing various herbs, and indeed these types of tonics have been used for centuries.

In this day and age it is important to use a powerful liver tonic that contains the most essential natural substances for healthy liver function. Such a powerful liver tonic is able to support the detoxification pathways in the liver which breakdown toxins. It is also able to improve the structural and functional integrity of the liver cells and liver filter.

Let us take a look at the various natural ingredients that need to be present in a liver tonic. This is available in a formula known as Livatone Plus which is a tonic that has been designed for today's world.

These are:-
- Glutamine
- Glycine
- Taurine
- Cysteine
- Vitamin C
- Vitamin E
- Natural Carotenoids
- Thiamine (Vitamin B1)
- Riboflavine (Vitamin B2)
- Nicotinamide (Vitamin B3)
- Calcium Pantothenate (Vitamin B5)
- Pyridoxine (Vitamin B6)
- Cyanocobalamin (Vitamin B12)
- Folic Acid
- Biotin
- Inositol
- Lecithin
- Zinc
- St Mary's Thistle (Milk Thistle)
- Cruciferous Vegetables
- Green Tea

For those who are interested, we will explain in detail, in the next few pages, how these individual ingredients work.

Amino Acids

Specific amino acids are essential for the liver to breakdown toxins and drugs and also for the efficient metabolism of nutrients by the liver.

Glutamine

This amino acid is required for phase two detoxification in the liver and is required in increased amounts by those who consume excessive alcohol. It is able to reduce the craving for alcohol. Glutamine supplementation is helpful for intestinal disorders such as peptic ulcers and leaky gut syndrome. Leaky gut is the term used to describe an inflamed condition of the lining of the bowel, which makes the bowel too permeable, so that toxins and incompletely digested food particles can be absorbed from the bowels directly into the liver. This increases the workload of the liver and may cause many health problems.

Glutamine is used as fuel by the brain and by the lymphocytes (white blood cells). It is essential for the lymphocytes to fight viruses such as hepatitis B and C.

Glutamine is converted in the body into glutamic acid, which, along with the amino acids cysteine and glycine, is converted into the powerful liver protector glutathione.

Glutathione is essential for liver phase two conjugation reactions used during detoxification of drugs and toxic chemicals.

Glutathione is a potent antioxidant that is produced in the healthy liver where it neutralizes oxygen molecules before they can damage cells. Glutathione is a component of the antioxidant enzyme glutathione-S-transferase, which is a widely acting liver-detoxifying enzyme. Indeed large amounts of glutathione are stored in the liver, where it detoxifies harmful compounds so they can then be excreted via the bile. Glutathione helps to reduce damage from cigarette smoke, alcohol, radiation, heavy metals, drugs and chemotherapy. Glutathione plays a vital role in preventing liver cancer. Glutathione levels decline with age, and this may accelerate the ageing process.

It is not worth taking glutathione supplements, as they are expensive and usually poorly absorbed. It is far more effective to increase glutathione levels by giving the liver, the raw materials it needs to make its own glutathione, namely, the amino acids glycine, glutamine and cysteine.

Glycine

This amino acid performs more biochemical functions than any other amino acids. It is required for the synthesis of bile salts, and is used by the liver to detoxify chemicals in the phase-two detoxification pathways.

Taurine

Inadequate levels of taurine are common in those patients with chemical sensitivities, allergies and poor diets. Taurine is the major amino acid required by the liver for the removal of toxic chemicals and metabolites from the body. Impaired body synthesis of taurine will reduce the ability of the liver to detoxify environmental chemicals such as chlorine, chlorite (bleach), aldehydes (produced from alcohol excess), alcohols, petroleum-based solvents and ammonia. Recent findings are demonstrating that taurine is one of the major nutrients involved in the body's detoxification of harmful substances and drugs, and should be considered in the treatment of all chemically sensitive patients. Taurine is helpful for fatty liver, high blood cholesterol and gall bladder problems, alcohol withdrawal, hepatitis and jaundice.

Taurine is a sulphur bearing amino acid that is present in all good liver tonics for very good reasons. It is required for the healthy production of bile, and the liver uses it to conjugate toxins and drugs to excrete through the bile. It helps the liver to excrete excessive cholesterol out of the body through the bile, and thus is an aid to weight control and cardiovascular health. Doses required can vary from 50 to 2000 mg daily. It is free of side effects but should not be taken on an empty stomach in those with stomach ulcers.

It is found in animal protein such as meat, seafood, eggs and dairy products but not in vegetable protein. Taurine is often deficient in strict vegans. Taurine regulates the transport of minerals across cell membranes and stabilises the electrical properties of cell membranes. For this reason, a deficiency of taurine has been linked to epileptic seizures, and combined with vitamin B 6, it has a useful anti-seizure effect in epileptics. It is made from two other amino acids methionine and cysteine.

Cysteine

Cysteine is an amino acid that contains sulphur, and is needed by the phase-two detoxification pathway. It is a precursor of glutathione, which is needed to breakdown pollutants and toxins and has powerful antioxidant effects. Aldehydes, which are toxic breakdown products of alcohol, rancid fats and smog, are partially neutralized by cysteine. A study reported that large doses of acetaldehyde (derived from alcohol), killed 90% of the mice that consumed it. A control group of mice were primed with vitamin C, vitamin B 1 and cysteine, and were then given the equivalent amount of acetaldehyde that had killed 90% of the other mice. None of the supplement-primed mice in the control group died.

Antioxidants

Antioxidants destroy free radicals and so help to detoxify and protect the cells of the body, including the liver cells, from toxins.

Vitamin C

Vitamin C is the most powerful antioxidant vitamin for the liver and reduces toxic damage to the liver cells from chemical overload. It neutralizes free radicals generated during the phase 1 detoxification pathway in the liver. Toxic chemicals are far less dangerous if there is plenty of vitamin C in the liver. It helps the liver to regulate cholesterol levels and improves immunity.

Vitamin E

Natural vitamin E is biologically more active than synthetic vitamin E. Vitamin E is a powerful antioxidant that protects fats from damage. Since cell membranes are composed of fats, vitamin E is the best protector of cell membranes. It does this by preventing free radicals from oxidizing cell membranes, which prevents them from becoming rancid. Thus vitamin E can help to protect the membranes surrounding liver cells. Vitamin E is also needed in those with a "fatty liver", where there is an accumulation of unhealthy oxidized fats in the liver cells.

Natural Carotenoids

Carotenoids such as betacarotene are most commonly found in fruits and vegetables and are most significant for human health. It is important to take only natural sources of beta-carotene and other carotenoids.

Beta-carotene gets converted in the body to vitamin A and yet has none of the toxic side effects of high doses of vitamin A. Large population studies have shown that low intakes of beta-carotene are associated with a higher incidence of cancer. Beta-carotene is a powerful protective antioxidant.

B Group Vitamins

Thiamine (Vitamin B 1)

This B vitamin has antioxidant properties and is helpful in reducing the toxic effects of alcohol, smoking and lead. Thiamine protects against many of the metabolic imbalances caused by alcohol. Deficiency of thiamine is common in those who consume excessive alcohol and this will often lead to poor mental function.

Riboflavine (Vitamin B 2)

This B vitamin is required during phase one detoxification in the liver, and is crucial in the production of body energy. Riboflavine deficiency is common in those who consume excessive alcohol and should be supplemented in such cases.

Nicotinamide (Vitamin B 3)

This is also known as Niacinamide, and is required by the liver's phase one detoxification system. It is needed for the metabolism of fats and helps to keep cholesterol levels under control.

Calcium Pantothenate (Vitamin B 5)

Several studies have found that pantothenate can lower cholesterol (by an average of 15%), and triglycerides (by an average of 30%) in those with elevated levels of these blood fats. A study showed that pantothenate speeds up liver detoxification of acetaldehyde after alcohol consumption. This is very important for those who consume excessive alcohol because acetaldehyde appears to be a major chemical in the toxic process that accompanies long term alcohol use. Pantothenate is required in increased amounts in liver disease and in those who use alcohol excessively.

Pyridoxine (Vitamin B 6)

Vitamin B 6 is required for effective phase one liver detoxification, and is essential for physical and mental health. Vitamin B 6 inhibits the formation of a toxic chemical called homocysteine, which accelerates cardiovascular disease.

Cyanocobalamin (Vitamin B 12)

Supplements of this powerful vitamin are essential for those who are strict vegetarians or those with nervous complaints. It is a great energizer of the nervous system and can reduce depression and fatigue. It is required for phase one detoxification of chemicals in the liver, and can help people who are allergic to sulphites, which are common food and wine additives.

A study showed that vitamin B 12 can effectively block most of the adverse reactions to sulphites such as hay fever, sinus, headache and bronchial spasms. B 12 is required for the liver to perform methylation, which inactivates the hormone oestrogen and enhances the flow of bile.

B 12 is required in increased amounts by those who use alcohol excessively, or in liver disease and pernicious anaemia.

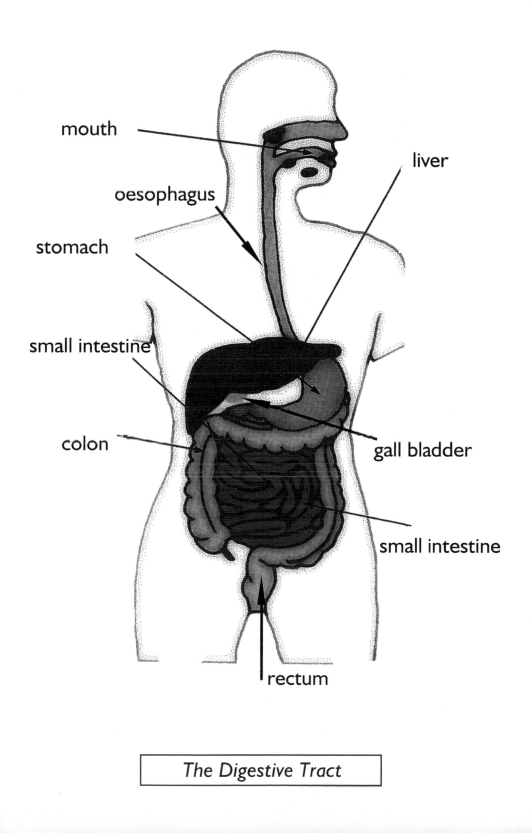

mouth

oesophagus

stomach

small intestine

colon

liver

gall bladder

small intestine

rectum

The Digestive Tract

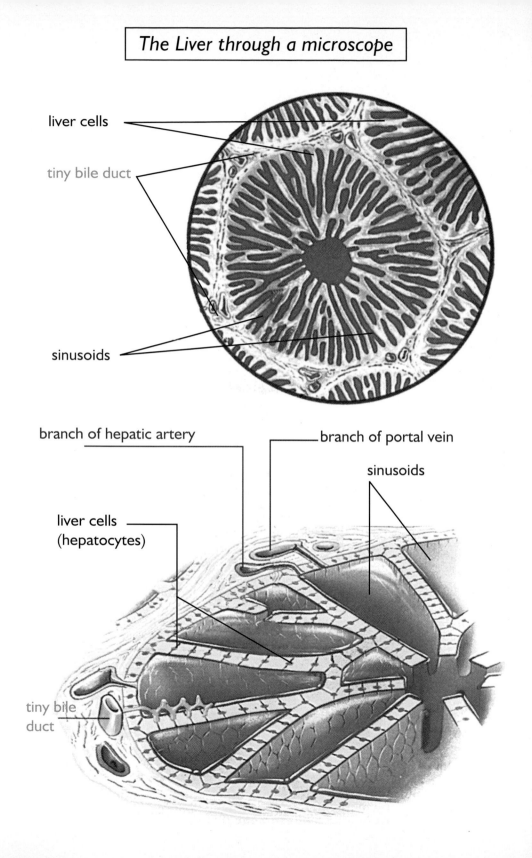

The Liver through a microscope

liver cells

tiny bile duct

sinusoids

branch of hepatic artery

branch of portal vein

sinusoids

liver cells
(hepatocytes)

tiny bile
duct

Folic Acid

Is required for the phase one detoxification pathway in the liver and for cell repair and division. There is an increased need in alcohol excess. Some studies have shown that folic acid exerts an anti-cancer effect.

Biotin

Biotin is one of the B vitamins and is produced in the intestines by friendly bacteria. It is found in foods such as nuts, whole grain foods, vegetables and brewer's yeast, and in supplement form. Liver cells that lack biotin will be deprived of the energy they need to detoxify chemicals and drugs.

Deficiency of this vitamin is not rare and can cause hair loss, dry flaky skin, rashes and fatigue. Those with a poor diet, alcoholism or long term antibiotic use, are at risk of deficiency.

Inositol

This vitamin is important in fat metabolism, and helps to remove fats from the liver. Deficiency of inositol can increase hardening of the arteries, increase blood cholesterol levels and lead to hair loss, constipation and mood swings. Excessive consumption of caffeine can reduce the level of inositol in the body.

Lecithin

Lecithin contains healthy fats, which are required for the functional and structural integrity of cell membranes. Lecithin is composed of the B vitamin choline, along with linoleic acid and inositol. A choline deficiency promotes liver damage and can be corrected with lecithin supplements. Choline has shown a protective effect against cirrhosis in animal studies. Trials are now being done to see if this protective effect can be reproduced in humans.

Lecithin is vital for fat metabolism and allows cholesterol to disperse in watery solutions so that it can be transported around the body to where it is needed, or removed from the body. This reduces the risk of fatty degeneration in arteries and vital organs. It can help those with the condition of fatty liver caused by incorrect diet or alcoholism.

Zinc

The mineral zinc has antioxidant properties and is part of the powerful antioxidant enzyme called superoxide dismutase (SOD). Zinc is vital for the efficient functioning of the cellular immune system needed to fight infections from viruses, parasites and fungal microorganisms.

St. Mary's Thistle (Milk Thistle)

Milk Thistle also known as "Silybum Marianum", is a herb with remarkable detoxifying and liver protective effects. It is a very well known liver herb, having been recommended in herbal texts since the late 1600's. Its most active constituent is silymarin, which is a bioflavonoid.

Research has shown that Milk Thistle can protect against some severe liver toxins. For example the poisonous mushroom "Amanita phalloides" leads to death in 40% of people who ingest it. This mushroom contains the toxins, phalloidin and amanitin, which are highly destructive to liver cells. Extracts of Milk Thistle containing the active ingredient silymarin, can protect the liver from phalloidin. Some animal experiments found that silymarin was 100% effective in preventing toxicity when given before poisoning by the mushrooms. Silymarin was also effective if given to the poisoned animals within 10 minutes after ingestion. Furthermore, if silymarin was given within 24 hours after ingestion it still prevented death, and greatly reduced the severity of liver damage. Silymarin also protects the liver in animals exposed to alcohol, and the solvent carbon tetrachloride.

Liver disorders in humans have been treated with silymarin with promising results. Patients with chronic hepatitis (liver inflammation) had improvements in liver function after taking silymarin for 3 months. Most liver toxins, including alcohol, produce damage to cell membranes via free radical generation. Silymarin functions as an antioxidant and reduces damage to cell membranes. It prevents the formation of leukotrienes, which are dangerous inflammatory chemicals produced by the immune system. Silymarin can increase the quantity of the powerful liver protector glutathione, and improves protein synthesis in the liver.

Cruciferous vegetables

Cruciferous vegetables such as broccoli, cauliflower, cabbage, Brussels sprouts, kale, bok choy, mustard greens and radish, contain important substances such as indoles, thiols and sulphur compounds, which enhance the liver's phase one and two detoxification pathways. Broccoli has a particularly good effect and enhances glutathione conjugation of toxins.

There is evidence that cruciferous vegetables are able to reduce the risk of cancer, and the American Cancer Society have been placing large advertisements in magazines with pictures of these vegetables, saying that "A defence against cancer can be cooked up in your kitchen. "

Green tea

Green tea exerts strong antioxidant actions and is also able to inhibit cancer cell growth. The Chinese, who are large drinkers of green tea, have a 60% less chance of oesophageal cancer. Parts of Japan where people drink a lot of green tea have a lower incidence of many types of cancers, including stomach, oesophageal and liver cancer.

Green tea may also be of benefit as an aid to weight loss through positive effects on fat and sugar metabolism.

All of the above ingredients are available finely ground and mixed together in either powder or capsule form in a formula called Livatone Plus.

This is far more practical, economical and convenient than having to take them all individually. The tonic can be taken in a dose of one teaspoon mixed in fresh juice just before meals, twice daily, or two capsules just before food, twice daily. Take this dosage for eight to twelve weeks. Then go on to a maintenance dose of one teaspoon daily, or two capsules daily, which can be continued for as long as needed. Some people find that they need to stay on a liver tonic in a maintenance dose permanently because of dysfunctional liver problems and the extra challenges faced by the liver in this day and age. Those who have a very dysfunctional liver, a fatty liver, or problems with excessive weight, can continue safely on the higher dose. Children over 3 years of age can take the powder in a reduced dosage of 1/4 to 1/3 of a teaspoon, mixed in fruit juice twice daily, before meals.

When beginning any liver tonic for the first time, always commence with a low dosage (say one quarter of the recommended dosage, eg. 1/2 a teaspoon of powder daily or 1 capsule daily), and stay on this low dose for the first week. Beginning with the maximum dose of a liver tonic may stimulate the liver's release of toxins too quickly, which could cause nausea, vomiting or headaches.

The Liver and Weight Loss

Vital Points for the Weight Conscious!

1.   The liver is the major fat burning organ in the body and regulates fat metabolism by a complicated set of biochemical pathways. The liver can also pump excessive fat out of the body through the bile into the small intestines. If the diet is high in fibre this unwanted fat will be carried out of the body via the bowel actions.

Thus the liver is a remarkable machine for keeping weight under control being both a fat burning organ and a fat pumping organ.

2.   If the diet is low in fibre, some of the fats (especially cholesterol) and toxins that have been pumped by the liver into the gut through the bile will recirculate back to the liver. This occurs via the entero-hepatic circulation. The term entero-hepatic circulation describes the recirculation of fluids (consisting mainly of bile acids) from the gut back to the liver. *See diagram on page 38*. The entero-hepatic circulation is very large, with approximately 95% of the bile acids being reabsorbed from the last section of the small intestine (ileum), into the portal vein to be carried back to the liver. The liver recirculates these bile acids back into the small intestines and the entire bile pool recycles through the entero-hepatic circulation six to eight times a day. If this recirculated fluid is high in fat and/or toxins, this will contribute to excessive weight.

A high fibre diet will reduce the recirculation of fat and toxins from the gut back to the liver. This is vitally important for those with excessive weight, toxicity problems and high cholesterol. The inclusion of plenty of raw fruits and vegetables as well as ground-up raw seeds will increase both soluble and insoluble fibre in the gut, and reduce recirculation of unwanted fat and toxins. Some people find that rice or wheat bran, psyllium husks and unprocessed homemade muesli can boost fibre efficiently.

3.   If the liver filter is damaged by toxins or clogged up (blocked) with excessive waste material it will be less able to remove small fat globules (chylomicrons) circulating in the blood stream. This will cause excessive fat to build up in the blood vessel walls. This fat may then gradually build up in many other parts of the body, including other organs, and in fatty deposits under the skin. Thus you may develop cellulite in the buttocks, thighs, arms and abdominal wall.

If the liver is dysfunctional, it will not manufacture adequate amounts of the good cholesterol (HDL), which travels out of the liver to scavenge the unhealthy cholesterol (LDL) from the blood vessel walls.

4.   If the liver filter is healthy it allows dietary cholesterol to be shunted into the liver for metabolism or excretion through the bile. A healthy liver filter is essential to properly regulate blood cholesterol levels. Poor liver function may increase your chances of cardiovascular diseases such as atherosclerosis, high blood pressure, heart attacks and strokes.

If the liver does not regulate fat metabolism efficiently, weight gain tends to occur around the abdominal area and a protuberant abdomen (potbelly) will develop. This is not good for the waistline! Another sign can be a roll of fat around the upper abdomen, which I affectionately call the "liver roll." This is often a sign of a fatty liver. It can be almost impossible to lose this abdominal fat until the liver function is improved. Once this is done the liver will start burning fat efficiently again and the weight comes off gradually and without too much effort from you. It is not necessary to make yourself miserable by following a low fat, low calorie diet. What is effective in the long term is to eat the correct foods and nutrients for the liver to improve its fat burning function. *(See principles of the diet on pages 20 to 28)*. A good liver tonic containing the liver herb St. Mary's Thistle, and sulphur containing amino acids will help the liver to burn fat more efficiently and thus is an aid to weight control.

5.   Many middle-aged people with excess fat in the abdominal area have a "fatty liver". In this condition the liver has stopped burning fat and has turned into a fat storing organ. It becomes enlarged and swollen with greasy deposits of fatty tissue. Those with a fatty liver will not be able to lose weight unless they first improve liver function, with a liver cleansing diet and a good liver tonic. If you have a fatty liver it is vital to be patient, as it can take between 3 to 12 months, depending upon the amount of fat deposited in the liver, to remove the excess fat from the liver. After this accumulated liver fat has been removed, weight loss will occur easily. If you have a very severe case of fatty liver it can take several years to lose all of the excessive weight.

However, this is very successful in the long term and provides the best chance of restoring your figure and your health. Fatty liver is common and doctors often tell their patients with this problem not to worry too much because it is not serious. I disagree with this, because if you have a fatty liver, your chances of high cholesterol, cardiovascular disease and mature-onset diabetes are significantly higher. Unfortunately, it is not uncommon to find a fatty liver in adolescents who consume a diet high in processed and fast foods.

Entero - hepatic circulation

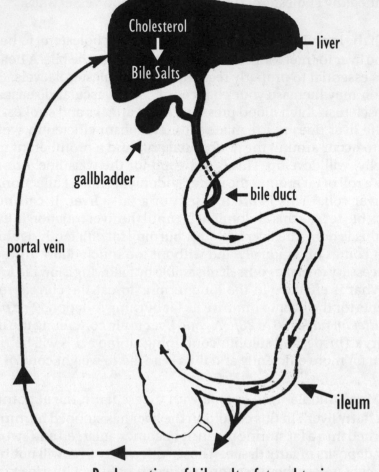

Cholesterol

↓

Bile Salts

← liver

gallbladder

← bile duct

portal vein

ileum

Reabsorption of bile salts, fat and toxins

6. If you overload the liver with the wrong type of hormone replacement therapy, drugs or toxins, the liver's biochemical pathways will have less energy reserves left over to perform their function of fat metabolism. Thus these things can lead to weight gain. For menopausal women with a weight problem, the best type of hormone replacement therapy is that which bypasses the liver, namely hormone patches, creams or buccal lozenges *(see page 52)*

Shopping and Grocery List
For Liver Lovers

Try to find a source of organically grown fruits and vegetables and organically raised free- range eggs and meats. This is not always possible in certain shopping centres and you can only do your best. Some supermarket chains have a great selection of healthy and/or organic products available. *See page 287* for information on organic supplies.

Some books give long lists of the specific fruits and vegetables that are most likely to be highly contaminated with insecticides. However, if you avoided all of these foods you would be missing out on valuable nutrients and also much pleasure. You can always try to purchase organically produced food, but please do not become highly stressed or anorexic if this is impossible all the time. It is important to support organic farming by increasing consumer demand for these products. This will help our internal and external environment, and protect the future for our children.

Shopping List
Raw and dried fruits of all varieties
Raw vegetables. Vegetables that are highly liver cleansing because of their high sulphur content are cruciferous vegetables (broccoli, Brussels sprouts, cabbage, cauliflower), garlic and onions.
Fruits and vegetables with deep bright pigments such as orange, yellow, red and green colors are very cleansing (eg. carrots, pumpkin, papaya, mangoes, berries, citrus fruits, red cabbage, purple cabbage, red and green capsicums).
Mushrooms - (field, shitake, button), potatoes, yams, avocado, olives, and seaweeds and sea vegetables (Kombu, Arame, Nori, Wakame)
Raw nuts - purchased raw and fresh, such as Brazil nuts, almonds, macadamias, cashews and walnuts, hazelnuts, pecans, and peanuts
Raw seeds - buy in small quantities and refrigerate. Flaxseed (linseed), sunflower, sesame, alfalfa, pumpkin seeds.

Rice and Grains - Wheat, cous cous, buckwheat, rye, barley, oats, quinoa, amaranth, spelt, kamut. Rice - brown, biodynamic, sweet, basmati, jasmin, glutinous, long grain, wild rice and white rice.

Legumes - These can be raw, cooked, canned (check out the packaged goods section for some ideas) or sprouted. The varieties are endless, try as many as you can as they are an essential source of protein and fibre. Green and yellow split peas, red and brown lentils, chick peas, broad beans, kidney beans, cannellini beans, black, azuki, mung, burlotti and butter are just a few.

Sprouts such as alfalfa, mung bean, broccoli sprouts, wheat grass, barley grass are a good source of chlorophyll, which is liver cleansing.

Breads - whole-grain, rye, rice, maize, multi-grain, stone ground, pita, sourdough and rice breads. Some wheat free breads that taste good are Wuppertaler, Pete and Vicky's, Demeter, Pav's and the Friendly Bakery.

Biscuits - crisp breads and crackers made from whole-grains, ie. corn and rice that are free of hydrogenated vegetable oils and fat. May be salt free or lightly salted. (Avoid sweet biscuits).

Pasta and Noodles - All kinds of pasta are available from the local supermarket, Asian grocery or health food store, including wheat free (rice, corn, potato and buckwheat). Try to buy pasta made from wholegrain. There are fresh rice noodles in different sizes which are quick and easy to use. Japanese noodles ie. Soba, buckwheat and Udon which are also very delicious

Meat - Chicken, preferably fresh and free range and don't forget to remove the skin. In fact all meat can be bought free range.

Eggs, preferably free range

Seafood - such as tuna, salmon, sardines, mackerel (oily fish), fresh fish fillets, shellfish. Canned fish is healthy. (Avoid eating seafood that is raw, smoked or deep-fried).

Spreads - for breads and biscuits such as hoummus, tahini, pesto, minced garlic with cold pressed oil and nut spreads (such as Brazil nut, cashew, peanut, almond). Miso and honey. Natural fruit jam, and fresh avocado is a great replacement for butter when using jam. Jams (sugarfree wherever possible) are available from your local supermarket or organic suppliers.

Oils - Cold pressed virgin vegetable and seed oils eg. Olive, flaxseed, safflower, sunflower, canola, peanut and grapeseed, etc.
To save money, try buying a large tin of oil and storing it under the sink away from heat and sunlight as you would potatoes! Then using a funnel pour it into a dark coloured glass bottle to keep handy. For salads use olive oil, linseed or canola. For Asian recipes use peanut or canola. For stir frying use olive oil, canola, sunflower or sesame. Later for variety try the taste of almond or avocado oil.

Beverages - soy milk, almond milk, oat milk, rice milk, water (filtered, distilled or purified), bottled or canned fruit and vegetable juices with no added sugar (check the labels for additives and sugar), tea (regular, green or herbal). Australia's Own Malt Free is great in tea - it has a similar texture to cows milk and coconut milk. Try using Carob as a flavouring instead of chocolate - it's yum!

Spices - chilli - whole and powder, ginger, coriander, cayenne, tumeric, basil, rosemary, fennel, oregano, sage, whole black pepper, cummin, cardamon is a favourite in all its forms, fenugreek, mustard, bay leaves, curry powder and leaves, clove powder and whole, cinnamon powder and sticks, nutmeg, allspice and others if they are natural.

Flour - Self raising and plain wholemeal, rye, soy, buckwheat, rice, chickpea (Besan), Kuzu (a starch made from the root of a Japanese plant - great for thickening soups, sauces, gravies etc) and maize flour (keep at least 3 varieties).

Sweeteners - Honey, pear and apple concentrate, maple syrup, sugar - raw, brown and palm , rice syrup, blackstrap molasses and dried fruit purée (most natural sweeteners can be obtained from your local health food store).

Other Seasonings and miscellaneous Items - Balsamic and apple cider vinegar, soy mayonaise, mustard, chilli sauce, tamari (a wheat free soy) fish sauce, shoyu, mirin, soy sauce, oyster sauce and any of your favourites. If you need a setting agent i.e to make jelly, try using Agar Agar (a combination of sea vegetables). Umboshi Plums are great for seasoning salads or used in cooking vegetables - they are quite salty and delicious.

Packaged Goods -

Canned fruit - in natural juice only, however poaching your own fruit is much more delicious.

Prepared stock - Campbells.

Canned beans - there are a couple of brands (Annalisa and Val Verdi) available in most local supermarkets that have no sugar or additives and have a large variety of beans to choose from.

Tinned tomatoes and paste - a good organic and cheap brand found in some supermarkets is 'Bioitalia.' Also check the no name brands, they often have just tomatoes and salt.

Tea of all kinds - try Formosan, Green and Jasmin, all delicious without milk.

'Orgran' which is found in most supermarkets - they make a delicious buckwheat pancake mix and many varieties of pasta.

'Vogel' make some designer breakfast cereals with a lot of variety.

'Arrowhead' and **'Nature's Path'** make some great adventurous cereals, including amaranth, kamut and corn flakes. There is also a delicious "coco pops" alternative. Most of these are organic. Keep an eye out!

Audrey's Tip for the first week

Choose 3 or 4 dishes from this book, then gradually add extra ingredients to your cupboard as you need them.

Fresh is best, especially for vegetables, salad items and fruit, so choose firm, clean (organic and/or in season where possible) produce, and refrigerate when necessary.

Only wash fruit and vegetables when you wish to use them as this stops them sweating and deteriorating.

Kitchen Utensils

Kitchen utensils needed to follow liver and bowel cleansing diet
Not all of these are essential but they will make working much easier and save you time!

Juice extracting machine for making fresh raw juices.
For juice ideas see page 168
Orange juice squeezer.
Coffee grinder, blender or food processor
Water filter or purifier.
Wok
Peeler, garlic press and grater
Spatulas - wooden, plastic + Slotted spoon, wooden spoon
Tongs and whisk
Non - Stick frying pan (stone coated is best)
Stainless steel fry pan and saucepans
Large firm chopping board
A set of measuring cups and spoons
Good quality sharp knives

Shop wisely with liver consciousness.

Love your liver and live longer!

Common Questions
Answered by Dr. Cabot

Q.   Where is my liver?

It is situated in the upper right abdominal and lower right thoracic area. This is known in medical terms as the right hypochondrium. The upper margin of the liver lies between the fifth and sixth ribs, and its lower margin can sometimes normally be felt below the right rib cage if you breath in deeply. In those with some forms of liver disease or fatty liver, the enlargement of the liver can easily be felt extending below the right rib cage. The liver is divided into a right and left section, which are called lobes. The liver is the largest and hardest working organ in the body.

The liver is such an important organ that it has two sources of blood supply, namely the hepatic artery and the portal vein. The portal vein drains the blood from the gastrointestinal tract and spleen, back to the liver, which is why we can say that the liver is the gateway to the body.

Q.   What can I do if I have Gallbladder Disease or Gallstones?

Diseases of the gall bladder and biliary system are surprisingly common, and many cases could be avoided simply by following the principles of the Liver Cleansing Diet *(see page 20 to 27)*.

The Liver and Gall Bladder Flush

The liver/gall bladder flush is a quick way of flushing toxins, fat, sludge and small gallstones out of the liver and gall bladder. It is becoming quite popular in Russia and the U.S.A.

I will warn you that it is not for the faint hearted, and can cause some unpleasant reactions. Quite a few people have told me of excellent results from this procedure, so you may find it of interest and also of help. This is particularly so if you have gallstones or sludge in the gall bladder, which may or may not cause discomfort. The presence of gallstones can be diagnosed from various imaging techniques such as an ultrasound scan,

CAT scan or cholecystogram. Many people have "silent gallstones" that do not trouble them and in such cases it is not necessary to panic and rush into surgery. Gallstones are often discovered accidentally when a patient is being investigated for some other problem. The natural history of these stones is that they will remain silent and cause no problems, and only around 18% of such stones will cause problems over a 15-year period. If you have stones that are not troubling you, I suggest that you follow the liver principles in this book and take a liver tonic and watch the stones slowly dissolve and shrink away.

If however the gall stones or sludge are causing upper abdominal pain, nausea, bouts of vomiting, pain in the right shoulder, or if there is a chance of infection or cancer in the gall bladder, then you must be guided by your own surgeon. Laparoscopic surgery (keyhole surgery) has made the recovery time after surgery to remove the gall bladder (cholecystectomy) much shorter. In some very acute biliary attacks, gall bladder removal can be life saving. However, remember this type of surgery can have risks and complications and nobody looks forward to an operation. Although complications from gall bladder surgery are not common, I have seen patients who have had more problems after cholecystectomy than they had before. These problems included leaking bile, damaged bile ducts, liver haemorrhage, recurrent pain and fatty liver. Indeed I have found that the incidence of fatty liver is higher after removal of the gall bladder. These are the reasons why some people opt to use the liver/gall bladder flush to try and avoid surgery. If you decide to do this please talk to your doctor first.

One evening I was giving a seminar in Florida, when a middle-aged gentleman stood up in front of several hundred people and proudly told his account of how he had flushed out his liver and gall bladder with olive oil and lemon juice. This had resulted in him passing 1425 small gallstones over several hours, which he had obviously gone to great lengths to count! These small stones had been eliminated from his body via his bowel actions.

For patients who believe that they need to stimulate the elimination of toxins and/or gall stones out of the bile ducts, a liver flush can be done to greatly increase the flow of bile through the liver and bile ducts.

A Standard Method
for the Liver and Gallbladder flush is:

1. Freshly squeeze some citrus fruits such as grapefruit, orange, lemon and limes to make 300 mls (11oz) of juice. This will have a slightly sour taste, which is good, as bitter tasting fruits and vegetables stimulate the flow of bile from the liver and gall bladder. Dilute this juice with 200 mls (7oz) of filtered water.

2. Finely grate 1 to 2 cloves of fresh garlic and half a teaspoon of fresh gingerroot, and then press both in a garlic press to make juice. Add this juice to the water and citrus juice mixture. Garlic and ginger are liver cleansing and garlic contains sulphur compounds that the liver requires for its detoxification enzymes.

3. Pour 300 mls (11oz) of cold pressed good quality olive oil into a warm glass.

4. Every 15 minutes swallow 3 tablespoons of the citrus juice mixture and 3 tablespoons of the olive oil. Try to relax in between these 15-minute intervals. Some people find it beneficial to lie down on their right side with a hot water bottle over the liver area, which helps to dilate the bile ducts to allow the passage of small stones and sludge from the gall bladder. Others prefer to sit in a warm bath, which also helps to dilate the bile ducts.

5. If you desire, collect all your bowel actions (they may be loose and messy) into a bucket and when the flush is over, place them in a large strainer or colander and run tap water over them. You will probably find many greenish stones/gritty sludge around the size of a lentil or slightly larger. There may also be some large soft stones full of fatty cholesterol. Some people may not want to collect their bowel actions and are content to hear the stones clanging as they land in the toilet bowl!

I recommend that a qualified health practitioner always supervises the liver/gallbladder flush.

Certain people such as pregnant women, young children, very elderly and frail people, insulin-dependent diabetics or those with severe liver disease or an acutely inflamed gallbladder, should not try the liver/ gallbladder flush and should discuss it with their own doctor.
Some people who do this flush may find that they feel very nauseated (bilious), and/or vomit several times. Abdominal cramps and diarrhoea may accompany this, before the stones are passed.

An Alternative Method for the Liver and Gallbladder flush is:

• Drink one quart (one litre) of organic unsweetened apple juice daily for five days. This will soften up the stones to such an extent that they can be squashed with the fingers. During these five days eat mainly raw fruits and vegetables and no dairy products, red meat or chicken.
• On the sixth day, skip dinner and at 6 p.m. take a tablespoonful of epsom salts with 3 glasses of water. Repeat this at 8 p.m.

- At 10 p.m. make a cocktail of 115ml (4 ounces) of olive oil and 115ml of fresh squeezed lemon juice. Shake this very well and drink immediately.
- Next morning you will pass green stones varying from the size of grains of sand to as large as your thumb nail. You may be amazed at the results, as have many thousands of people who have used this technique to avoid surgery.

Preparation for the flush:

To prepare for the flushing procedure, I recommend that during the two days prior to the commencement of the flush, you only consume raw fruits and vegetables and drink 2 litres (4 pints) of water daily. This preparation will lessen the chance of a bad reaction.

Begin the liver flush in the morning after some brisk walking and deep breathing exercises. Make sure that you drink two litres of water gradually by sipping it slowly during the day, otherwise the flush may induce dehydration.

Some protagonists of this procedure, recommend that you begin the flush at 7 p.m. because they believe that the gall bladder is "more active at night". This may be true, however you will not get much sleep that night, if you decide to do the flush while the moon is shining!

If you are a person who forms recurrent gall stones you can do this flush 3 times every year to prevent gall stones from building up. Some people do it every month and find that it does not cause any problems or side effects. If you follow the principles of the liver cleansing diet found in this book, you should not have to do this procedure very often, if at all. This is because a healthy liver manufactures and secretes healthy bile, which prevents gall bladder inflammation and gallstones.

We do know that family history often plays a part in liver and gall bladder disease so if you find yourself with gallstones, have a good look at your family history and take extra special care of your liver. Gallstones are more common during pregnancy. If gallstones are recurrent in younger persons, this may be a sign of an underlying blood disease.

Other Treatments

Other treatments available for gall stones consist of drugs used to dissolve the stones. This is not hugely successful because it takes 6 months - 2 years for the stones to dissolve and the recurrence rate is high. Only stones made from cholesterol can be dissolved with drugs such as the bile acids chenodeoxycholic acid and ursodeoxycholic acid. These drugs will not dissolve calcified stones, which makes only around 10% of patients with gallstones suitable candidates for these drugs. Therefore these drugs are not recommended for the majority of patients with gallstones.

Gall bladder disease is very common, with around one million new cases of gallstones occurring every year in the U.S.A. This equates to 1 in every 250 persons who develop gallbladder problems annually, and the incidence is only slightly less in Australia. So do not feel alone if you have this problem! The good news is that most cases of gall bladder disease could be prevented if we consumed a diet that was good for the liver.

Q. What Herbal Teas are good for Liver and Bowel Cleansing?

Good cleansing herbs to choose from are fennel, dandelion root, gingerroot, chamomile, burdock root, peppermint, fenugreek, red clover, cleavers, chickweed and nettle.

An infusion is best for leaves, flowers and other light parts of a plant. This is made by bringing water to a boil, taking it off the heat, adding the herbs, and then covering the pot and leaving the mixture to steep for 15 to 20 minutes. Strain and drink when warm, and if desired sweeten with a small amount of honey. For herbal infusions the general ratio of herbs to water is 1:20 (eg. one ounce of herbs to 20 ounces of water).

A decoction is best for heavier parts of plants such as bark, roots or seeds. To make a decoction simmer the herbs in filtered water for 30 to 60 minutes. Strain and drink when warm, and sweeten with a small amount of honey if desired. For decoctions the general ratio of herbs to water is 1:10. These ratios are general guidelines and may be varied considerably by your herbalist.

It is preferable to make herbal teas in glass, ceramic, stainless steel or clay pots. Aluminium or Teflon coated saucepans should not be used.

fresh ginger tea

500mls (1 pint) water

2-inch slice	fresh ginger root
1	lemon
4	cloves
1 stick	cinnamon

Dash nutmeg or cardamom

Pass ginger through juicer and squeeze in lemon juice.
Place this in saucepan, add water, cloves and cinnamon.
Simmer for 15 minutes and add nutmeg or cardamom.
You may sweeten with a little honey or raw sugar if desired.

Q. What is the difference between Livatone and Livatone Plus?

Livatone

Livatone is a natural liver tonic containing the liver herbs St Mary's Thistle, Globe artichoke and Dandelion, combined with the amino acid taurine, and lecithin. It also contains natural sources of chlorophyll, carotenoids and fibre. It is available in capsule and powder form.

Livatone can be used as a general liver tonic and its benefits include:
An aid to weight loss and fat burning
An aid for those with high blood levels of cholesterol and triglycerides
Reduction of fluid retention and irritable bowel syndrome
As a fibre supplement to reduce constipation and bloating (especially the powder form)
An aid for digestive problems and gall bladder dysfunction

Livatone can be taken by anyone wanting to generally improve the function of their liver, which is a good idea from time to time considering that the liver is the most important organ in the body, and in this day and age is in need of support.

Livatone can be used by people of all ages, including children over 2 years of age. Children under 10 years of age should use the powder dissolved in fruit juice before meals in a dose of 1/4 to 1/3 of a teaspoon twice daily. The dose for adults and children over 10 years of age is one teaspoon of powder twice daily stirred into juice just before meals, or 2 capsules twice daily with water just before meals.

Livatone Plus

Livatone Plus has a very different formula to Livatone, and can be described as a more powerful formula for metabolic problems or dysfunctions of the liver.

Livatone Plus contains the liver herb St Mary's Thistle, combined with sulphur bearing amino acids Taurine, Glycine, Cysteine and Glutamine. Livatone Plus also contains all the important B vitamins and lipotrophic cofactors such as Inositol, Folic acid and Biotin. It contains antioxidants to reduce liver damage and inflammation, such as Green Tea, vitamins C, E and natural betacarotene. It also contains lecithin and broccoli powder to help liver function.

Livatone Plus contains the essential nutrients to support the phase one and two detoxification pathways in the liver.

Livatone Plus is beneficial in the following conditions:

• Poor detoxification capability in the liver. These people often have multiple chemical, drug and food sensitivity. They may have been exposed to liver toxins. These people often have Chronic Fatigue Syndrome.

• Those who work in high-risk occupations which expose them to a high load of potential liver toxins such as petrochemicals, insecticides and solvents. For example painters, hair-dressers, motor mechanics, agricultural workers, foundry workers, plumbers, plant and transport operators, those in the dry cleaning industry, and some process and factory workers. If such workers support the liver with protective supplements they will reduce the risk of liver damage. Safe work practises are also of vital importance to minimise risk of contact exposure.

• Chronic headaches (including migraines) associated with nausea, especially if analgesic use is high.

• Those with skin problems such as inflammatory rashes, itchy skin and brown liver spots.

• Those with unstable blood sugar levels such as hypoglycaemia. These people often have strong sugar cravings and great difficulty sticking to a long-term healthy diet. Unstable blood sugar levels are known as glucose intolerance and this is often a forerunner to Type 11 diabetes. Type 11 diabetes is often associated with obesity and a fatty liver. Livatone Plus helps to stabilise blood sugar levels and makes it much easier to resist sugar cravings and stick to a healthy diet.

• Liver damage from various causes such as:

Viral infections of the liver with hepatitis A, B and C, glandular fever and other chronic viral infections that attack the liver.

Liver inflammation (hepatitis) from toxins, alcohol excess, recreational drugs, analgesic excess and drug induced hepatitis.

Autoimmune liver diseases such as Sclerosing Cholangitis, Primary Biliary Cirrhosis, Chronic Active Hepatitis or connective tissue diseases.

Fatty liver induced by incorrect diet, alcohol or diabetes.

Cirrhosis (scarring) of the liver from multiple causes.

Nodular hyperplasia of the liver

Liver cysts

Gall bladder dysfunction and gallstones.

Livatone Plus is available in capsule and powder form. The regular dosage in adults is one-teaspoon twice daily stirred into a nice fresh juice just before meals, or 2 capsules twice daily with water just before meals. In children over 2 years of age, Livatone Plus can be used to improve liver function in the above complaints. The dosage for children under 10 years of age is 1/4 to 1/3 of a teaspoon twice daily in fruit juice. Children under 10 find it difficult to swallow capsules and the powder should be used.

Both types of Livatone can be taken long term, as they are all natural products and free of side effects. The occasional person is allergic to psyllium, which is found in Livatone, in which case Livatone Plus should be used. Rarely there may be such a severe allergy to salicylates that the person is unable to take any herbs. Most herbs and plants contain salicylates *(see page 160)*. If salicylate allergy is severe you will have to avoid all products containing herbs and rely on vitamins and amino acids taken individually.

After taking **Livatone** or **Livatone Plus** for 2 - 3 months you can go onto a maintenance dose which is two capsules daily or one teaspoon daily. This can be continued indefinitely if you so desire, particularly if you feel healthier while taking **Livatone** formulas.

When starting any liver tonic it is important to begin with a reduced dose to avoid any strong reactions. These can occur because your liver is eliminating toxins rapidly for the first time in years, or rarely because you may be allergic to one of the ingredients. Beginning doses for both types of **Livatone** are 1/2 a teaspoon daily or one capsule daily. Take this dose for one week and if you continue to feel well you may go up to the regular dose on the second week. The regular dose is two capsules twice daily or one teaspoon twice daily.

Q. How can I Boost my Immune System Naturally?

If you or your family members are always "coming down with something", and always trying to fight off infections with antibiotic or antifungal drugs, then you really need to look at nutritional medicine as an effective preventative weapon.

*If your immune system is overburdened you may have
the following problems.*

- Chronic or recurrent viral infections, especially glandular fever (Epstein Barr Virus)
- Swollen glands
- Recurrent Herpes (genital or cold sores)
- Frequent skin infections
- Frequent inflammation and/or infections in the upper respiratory tract eg. sinuses, nose, ears or throat
- Recurrent bronchitis
- Recurrent cystitis
- Recurrent fungal and yeast infections such as candida and tinea
- Unhealthy bacteria and parasites in the bowel (dysbiosis)

Do you really want to put up with these things for much longer?
Do you want to rely upon the long-term use of antibiotics and other drugs that may be toxic to the liver, kidneys and immune system?

Such drugs usually become increasingly ineffective with long-term use, and often breed resistant and unhealthy microorganisms in the body.

A natural plan to fight these infections for people of all ages consists of

• Follow the principles of the Liver Cleansing Diet *(see page 20 to 27)*. This is vitally important because the liver reduces the workload of the immune system, and allows it to rest and become stronger. You may also need a liver tonic.

• Take Olive Leaf Extract (500mg) capsules, one capsule, two or three times daily just before food. Children can take Olive Leaf Elixir. Olive leaf extract has been used as a natural antibiotic for thousands of years, but it is only recently that scientific research has shown that its active ingredient *oleuropein*, has the ability to fight a broad range of infective microorganisms. Oleuropein has been found to be effective in fighting bacteria, fungi, yeasts, parasites and viruses in laboratory studies. **Ref 10**

• Take anti-oxidants, which help your white blood cells to kill microorganisms. The most important anti-oxidants for this purpose are Vitamin C, Vitamin D and Vitamin A (or betacarotene). Cod liver oil is a good source of the fat-soluble anti-oxidants and can be obtained in liquid or capsule form.

• Ensure adequate intake of the minerals required by the immune system to fight infections. These are zinc, magnesium and selenium. A good source of these minerals is found in Selenium Designer Yeast Powders, which can be stirred into fresh juices. Take 2 teaspoons of powder daily.

• Drink herbal teas such as Golden Seal, Green tea and Echinacea, which can be sweetened with lemon and honey or raw sugar if desired.

• Eat foods and condiments that are natural antibiotics; raw garlic, onions, leeks, shallots, radishes, fenugreek, fresh gingerroot, chilli and plenty of raw salads and fruits and their juices. Some people find it difficult to eat hot spicy things because they have a very sensitive digestive system. Always make sure that you have hot spicy things with plenty of food, and even small amounts of these things can help to expel infected mucous from your body. There are several ways to eat raw garlic. You can grate it, expel its juice in a garlic press or chop it into tiny pieces. These forms of garlic can be mixed well into cooked foods and salads and in this form are easy to tolerate. This is especially good for children with recurrent infections and if you do not tell them about it, they probably will not know they are eating it. You can also add some garlic juice to your vegetable juice cocktail. Raw garlic and other plants from the onion family are superb powerful natural antibiotics and can help to eradicate and control infections from any part of the body, even in cases where there is resistance to antibiotic drugs. If you absolutely hate raw garlic and its odour, then you will have to rely upon garlic capsules, which are not as effective.

• Avoid mucous-producing foods such as dairy products, margarines, processed and preserved foods (especially processed meats).

Q. What Hormone Replacement Therapy (HRT) is best for the Liver?

All drugs, including natural hormones must eventually pass through the liver, where they are filtered out of the blood stream and broken down (metabolised) into forms that can be eliminated from the body via the bile or urine. Hormone Replacement Therapy (HRT) that is taken in a tablet (oral) form, will be absorbed from the intestines and pass immediately through the liver via the liver's portal circulation of blood. Thus the liver may breakdown a large portion of the hormone dose before it can get into the general circulation to be carried to the body cells. This is why higher doses of hormones are required if they are administered in tablet form. In many people this does not cause any problems, whereas in others the liver may either render the hormones ineffective or become overworked by the task of breaking down the hormones. In the latter case, side effects such as weight gain, fluid retention, nausea, headaches, high blood pressure or even blood clots may result. In such cases it is best to stop the hormone therapy or change to another form of hormone therapy which is not absorbed from the intestines into the liver.

It is easy to administer natural hormones in forms that are absorbed directly into the blood circulation before they get to the liver. This enables smaller doses to be used because the hormones have a chance to perform their function on the body cells before the liver breaks them down. Suitable forms of hormones to achieve this effect are hormone patches, creams or lozenges (sometimes called by the French name of troches). Patches and creams are absorbed very well across the skin into the small blood vessels found in the subcutaneous layer of the skin. Patches are available containing natural oestrogen or natural oestrogen plus progestogen. Hormone creams give more flexibility because they can be tailor made to suit the individual, and can be compounded to include any variety of natural hormones such as the three different types of natural oestrogen (oestradiol, oestrone and oestriol), natural progesterone, testosterone and DHEA. It is also easier to adjust doses of hormones up or down in such creams. Generally half a teaspoon of the cream is used and massaged into the skin of the inner upper thigh twice daily. The skin must be dry and the cream must be massaged deeply into the skin. In those who are overly sensitive to hormones or have medical problems, we can use very small and therefore very safe doses of hormones in cream form. This is a breakthrough for women with medical problems who have been told that they can never enjoy the benefits of natural hormone replacement therapy.

The hormonal lozenges are placed between the upper gum and the cheek, and left to slowly dissolve into the small blood vessels under the surface of the mucous membrane of the cheek. They must not be chewed, sucked or swallowed, otherwise they will end up in the intestines and pass straight through the liver. The doses used in the lozenges are generally higher than those used in the creams. The lozenges can be tailor made to suit the individual, using any possible combination, and amounts of natural hormones such as oestradiol, progesterone, testosterone and DHEA.

I have been treating women with hormonal problems since the mid 1970s, and have seen many trends and fashions in hormonal replacement therapy come and go. The most important thing that I have learnt, is that every woman is an individual and needs fine-tuning to balance her unique hormonal and metabolic characteristics. You do not learn this from textbooks but from seeing thousands of women over many years who have often tried many other avenues of help. Some women require much higher doses and wider varieties of hormones than do others, although I always like to start with the smallest necessary dose. Initial prescriptions and follow up adjustments to dosage must be guided by measuring the level of hormones in the blood. These blood tests are very accurate. I prefer using blood tests to salivary hormone tests, although those experienced with the latter may find them of use.

When choosing Hormone Replacement Therapy (HRT), your Body Type needs to be taken into consideration - are you Android, Gynaeoid, Thyroid or Lymphatic. *See diagram on page 93.*

Android women and men tend to put on weight in the upper part of their body, especially around the midriff, and may develop a pot belly and a roll of fat around the liver. I call this the "liver roll." *See diagram on page 18* . Fatty liver is more common in Android shapes and makes it difficult for them to lose weight. Because their liver is often dysfunctional they do not tolerate large doses of hormones. Furthermore they do not need large doses, because they still produce significant amounts of hormones from their fat and adrenal glands after the ovaries shut down at menopause. After menopause they tend to produce plenty of male hormones such as DHEA and testosterone from their adrenal glands, and their bone density is usually good. Although I am generalising, I would tend to use small doses of natural oestrogens and progesterone in the form of creams for Android women. This is because this form of HRT does not stress the liver and will not cause weight gain and side effects. Furthermore it is easy to fine-tune the doses of hormones up or down in these hormonal creams.

Gynaeoid women have wide curvaceous hips, and tend to put on weight in the oestrogen dependent areas of the body such as the hips, lower buttocks and thighs and may get cellulite in these areas. They tend to be oestrogen dominant and need more progesterone than any other hormones. I would tend to use only small doses of natural oestrogen, and larger doses of natural progesterone in the form of lozenges or creams.

Thyroid body types are fine boned with long and lean limbs and may have an earlier than average menopause. They do not produce significant levels of steroid sex hormones during the postmenopausal years and may have severe symptoms of menopause. Their bone density tends to be low and osteoporosis is a concern in these very fine boned women. They often need higher doses of a wider range of hormones such as testosterone, DHEA, oestrogen and progesterone. Creams may not be strong enough and they may prefer lozenges or even implants or injections.

Lymphatic body types are the opposite of the thyroid types, in that they put on weight very easily. This weight is distributed all over their body so that they have thick puffy limbs. They have a dysfunctional lymphatic system, which causes fluid retention and bloating. They really need to follow a dairy free diet, and do regular exercise to control their weight and fluid excess. I would tend to use hormonal creams in lymphatic body types because they do not aggravate fluid retention. Lymphatic types can use natural diuretics such as garlic, ginger, parsley and the herbs dandelion and uva ursi, to promote the elimination of excessive fluid. For more detail on body types read my book titled "The Body Shaping Diet."

For more information on tailor made
Hormone Replacement Therapy call the Hormonal Advisory Service
on (02) 4653 1445 or (02) 9387 8111.

Q. Can I Cook with Oil on the Liver Cleansing Diet?

Did you know that low fat diets are often very boring and difficult to stick to for more than several weeks because they do not produce a feeling of satisfaction after eating. You will be more successful if you follow the "right fat diet" and not a "low fat diet". Oils used for cooking should be cold pressed varieties of vegetable and seed oils. They should be fresh, and stored in a cool place (refrigerator is best) away from the light to prevent the oils from becoming rancid. If possible buy and store oils in dark coloured glass bottles because light is more damaging to oils than contact with air. Unfortunately you will still find the majority of bottled oils in supermarkets are stored in transparent plastic containers. The mono-unsaturated oils such as extra virgin olive oil, sunflower oil and canola oil are suitable for salad dressings. Flaxseed oil can also be used for salad dressings and has a sweet nutty flavour.

Any oil can be damaged (oxidised) by frying it at very high temperatures. Saturated oils are more resistant to damage caused by free radicals generated during oxidation at high temperatures. Therefore saturated oils such as coconut and palm oils can also be used for stir-frying as can olive oil.

All oils are fragile and susceptible to damage, however some more so than others. Olive oil is reasonably stable and will generally last for 2 years after it is manufactured. Canola oil, sunflower oil and pumpkin seed oil will last around one year after manufacturing. Flaxseed (linseed) oil has excellent health benefits but should be consumed quickly because if storage conditions are not carefully controlled it lasts only three months, and sometimes much less after manufacturing. For these reasons it is best to buy small quantities of these oils, store them meticulously and consume them within a few weeks.

You should never use frying oils more than once, because toxic substances and free radicals will build up in these refried oils. The large vats of oils used in fast food restaurants to repeatedly fry chips and fish etc. is very toxic for the body. These vats may use the same reheated oils for many days and become more and more unhealthy.

The best way to use oils in cooking is to follow the Chinese tradition, which is not surprising, as the Chinese understand the effect of cooking methods upon liver function. The Chinese begin the cooking process by adding water, soy sauce or vegetable sauces to the wok and gradually heat it before adding any oil. They often add the foods to be cooked, such as vegetables, seafood or meat before adding any oil. They take care not to let the temperature of the oil rise above 170°F(77 °C) which is best achieved by heating gradually and slowly. The temperature of 170°F is approximately the temperature at which oils start to rapidly breakdown and oxidise.

Similar principles apply to baking foods with oils, taking care not to overheat the food. You may use olive oil, coconut oil or palm oil for baking.

Q. Why should I use Cold Pressed Oils instead of Hydrogenated Oils?

Cold pressed oils contain their component essential fatty acids in their natural state of "Cis" fatty acids, which are a curly flexible shape, and this is why the oils remain liquid. These cis - fatty acids are the correct shape for your cell membranes and fit very well into your cellular structure.

The manufacturing process of hydrogenation electrically converts the chemical structure of cis-fatty acids to trans-fatty acids. Trans- fatty acids are a different shape- they are straight and rigid and they do not fit nicely into your cell membranes. Indeed they can be described as social misfits in cellular society- inorganic aliens if you like.

Toxic trans-fatty acids have the following disadvantages:

They are harder to absorb from the gut and are not as nutritious.
They increase platelet stickiness, which increases the risk of blood clots.
They interfere with cell membrane function slowing down metabolism and increasing weight gain.

The liver cells do not like trans-fatty acids and do not know how to handle them, so they may accumulate in the liver. People who eat a lot of trans-fatty acids will often develop a fatty liver and elevated cholesterol.

Medical studies show that a high intake of trans-fatty acids can increase cholesterol and triglyceride levels. Animal studies suggest that a high intake of trans-fatty acids will increase the size of fatty plaques inside the arteries.

During the process of hydrogenation, hydrogen bubbles are passed through the oil which partially converts the polyunsaturated oil into saturated oil. This process was first achieved in 1940 and produced the first popular brand of cooking oil. Many of today's experts on oils believe that if the process of hydrogenation was just discovered it would not be developed and used by commercial oil producers. There would be just too much bad publicity. There are a small number of oils that are naturally hydrogenated, such as palm and coconut oils, which are suitable for stir frying because of their increased stability. These naturally hydrogenated oils are also used for chocolate production. Thankfully, naturally hydrogenated oils are healthier than processed hydrogenated oils and it is fine for you to consume them in small quantities.

Processed hydrogenated oils

These oils are found in margarine, hydrogenated vegetable oils (many of the pale coloured oils in plastic bottles in supermarkets), and processed foods such as cakes and biscuits made with hydrogenated vegetable oils. Look on the labels of biscuits and cakes and you will see hydrogenated oils, in many brands. Obviously it is impossible to completely avoid consuming any hydrogenated oils, and indeed a small amount will not harm you at all. Those who consume large amounts of hydrogenated oils regularly (and particularly if they are lacking the good quality essential fatty acids), may suffer with adverse health consequences.

Q. How much Alcohol can I Drink?

It is not necessary to be a "teetotaller" and exclude alcohol, unless you have liver disease, when your liver specialist must guide you. A liver specialist is called a hepatologist and is a type of physician.

I recommend that you have no more than two to three glasses of alcohol in any 24-hour period. It is also prudent to have days where you do not drink any alcohol, and confine drinking to three days in any one week. This gives your liver plenty of time to eliminate the waste products of alcohol metabolism. A good liver tonic can also help the liver to metabolise alcohol and will often reduce the symptoms of a hangover.

Excessive alcohol, like any liver toxin, can decrease the rate of metabolism and secretion of fat in the bile, leading to a fatty liver. Long term use of excessive alcohol is very toxic to many parts of the body. Alcohol excess can damage the brain cells, causing dementia and nerve damage resulting in a clumsy uncoordinated gait. It can damage the liver and pancreas causing liver scarring (cirrhosis) and diabetes. Alcohol and cirrhosis are a game of risk. Not all severe alcoholics get cirrhosis, while some social drinkers do. Women are more likely to get alcoholic cirrhosis because they do not breakdown alcohol as efficiently as men.

Q. Can I drink Coffee and Tea on the Liver Cleansing Diet?

The best way to consider coffee and other beverages high in caffeine is as an occasional treat rather than a habit. Like nicotine and alcohol, caffeine is potentially addictive or habit forming, and this is seen in the unpleasant withdrawal symptoms that occur after eliminating coffee in those who consume large amounts regularly. Caffeine may exacerbate the cramps and diarrhoea common in irritable bowel syndrome. Heavy use of caffeine (say more than 6 cups daily), may produce stomach inflammation and aggravate stomach ulcers by causing an increased secretion of stomach acid. Caffeine relaxes the valve between the oesophagus and the stomach, which can allow acid stomach contents to reflux up into the oesophagus. This can lead to heartburn and indigestion. Even decaffeinated coffee can cause digestive problems because, like strong tea, it contains tannic acid which can aggravate the stomach.

It is best to keep your consumption of coffee down to one to two cups daily. If you have digestive problems and IBS you may need to eliminate it all together. Strong tea can be an intestinal irritant just like coffee and should not be drunk regularly. Very weak tea and even better, herbal teas are much easier on the mucosal lining of the stomach. Some people drink their tea and coffee with cow's milk and over the course of a day may be consuming a large amount of cow's milk. It could be the cow's milk that is upsetting your digestive tract rather than the coffee or tea. I think that soymilk tastes quite nice in ordinary tea, and some people enjoy it with instant or plunger coffee. This is a personal thing and some people enjoy "soychinos" instead of cappuchinos.

Q. How much Fresh Juice should I drink?

This is an individual thing because some people love raw juices while others cannot stand them. Generally speaking, for the average healthy person who is trying to improve liver function, one medium sized glass of juice daily is sufficient. If you do not enjoy juices you do not have to make them and you may simply eat lots of raw fruits and vegetables instead. Diabetics are advised to avoid juices containing sugar, such as all fruit juices and carrot juice, and confine themselves to juices made with green vegetables and their leaves.

See page 168, for some delicious healthy juice suggestions

Q. How can I follow the Liver Cleansing Diet when Eating Out?

This can be achieved with a little planning and forethought on your part, which is more important if you suffer with food allergies, food intolerances or irritable bowel syndrome. Avoid drinking alcohol on an empty stomach and do not mix your drinks. Sip the alcohol slowly and alternate it with still water.

Let the restaurant or hostess know ahead of time that you will want to avoid certain foods, and this can allow them the time to prepare specific dishes and also avoids a fuss at the table. Advise them that you want to avoid preservatives and additives such as MSG and don't forget to be assertive as you will be the one who will suffer later! If the hostess insists that you try a food that you know will upset you or completely blow your diet, insist that you will be perfectly happy to eat the other delicious things that she has prepared and that you do not feel deprived at all.

If you want to avoid dairy products you will find that Italian and Asian restaurants have many dairy free dishes on their menus. They usually use coconut milk or tomato sauces instead of dairy creamy sauces. Always order a nice fresh salad, and specify that you do not want commercial salad dressings but require olive oil, organic vinegars or lemon if these things suit you. A safe desert is fruit salad or fruit sorbet. Some types of puddings made with fresh ingredients may be easy to digest. If you suffer with gas and indigestion do not forget to take your enzyme tablets and liver tonic with you to the restaurant or party.

Q.   Must I avoid Eggs and Coconut on the Liver Cleansing Diet?

Eggs are very high in cholesterol and if we listen to some nutritionists and the popular press we usually find that eggs are portrayed as dangerous and unhealthy, especially for those with heart problems. I do not agree with the general opinion that eggs should be considered suspect, because eggs contain high concentrations of many valuable nutrients. Moreover most of the studies that showed eggs raise cholesterol were done using powdered eggs. Powdered eggs contain oxidised or damaged cholesterol known as oxy-cholesterol, and this has a different effect in the body than pure fresh cholesterol. Other studies have found that hard-boiled eggs do not raise cholesterol levels in the majority of patients. A study done at the University of California found that the consumption of two boiled eggs daily did not increase cholesterol levels. The reason why eggs consumed in moderation is health promoting, is that eggs have a high content of lecithin. Lecithin has been proven to lower cholesterol and helps to keep it soluble so that it does not form plaques in the blood vessels. Eggs are also high in the sulphur bearing amino acids taurine, cysteine and methionine, which are required by the liver to regulate bile production, detoxification and cholesterol levels.

Eggs are only healthy if they are cooked correctly, and the best way to eat them is poached or boiled (soft or hard-boiled is OK). Never fry eggs and only use fresh eggs. Try not to break the egg yolk while cooking the eggs because air and light will begin to oxidise the egg's cholesterol. Of course you do not need to become paranoid, as this does not happen within a few minutes.

Generally speaking I would say limit the ingestion of eggs to no more than 10 to 12 per week, however this is an individual thing. If you have very high cholesterol you should ask your doctor to guide you, however I do not believe that you must avoid all eggs. Ask your doctor to do a fasting blood test to check the effect of eating eggs in your particular case. This way you can be sure and prove what effect they have. Remember that everyone is an individual with unique hormonal and metabolic differences, and nutritional medicine takes this into account.

Coconut is another much maligned food and indeed is unworthy of its jaded reputation. I personally prefer Asian sauces, especially delicious Thai recipes, which are made with coconut milk or coconut cream, to creamy sauces made with dairy products. I find that coconut milk and/or cream sauces are light, and do not produce mucous in the body. I have never found that fresh coconut, coconut milk or coconut sauces have caused high cholesterol levels or weight problems in my patients. If you have a fatty liver it is important not to overindulge in any fat and this is just common sense. Simply consume a sensible and satisfying amount of these foods, and make sure that they are fresh so that their contained fats are not oxidised.

Remember that the liver makes 80% of the body's cholesterol and cholesterol levels are regulated automatically by a HEALTHY liver. If you consume a little more cholesterol on one day, the liver will not manufacture as much of its own cholesterol and things will balance out nicely. Liver function has a much greater effect upon cholesterol levels than does a modest consumption of healthy foods containing cholesterol.

Q. Why is the Liver and Bowel Cleansing Diet Dairy Free?

I have purposely excluded all dairy products from the recipes in this book because of my personal beliefs and experiences and also because of the influence of several books I have read on the subject of cow's milk. My dietary and culinary philosophies are not conventional as far as many dieticians, nutritionists or doctors are concerned, and may not be agreed with or accepted by all. I have found that everyone is different, with unique hormonal and metabolic characteristics, which means that some people will have individual intolerances or idiosyncratic reactions to foods. This means that some trial and error will be involved in finding the best diet for oneself. Some people are able to consume dairy products with no problems.

Others will have problems from eating dairy products, such as recurrent infections of the respiratory tract, sinuses, ears and skin, mucous excess, different types of allergic reactions, asthma, and irritable bowel. I believe that in some people, dairy products may aggravate autoimmune diseases such as lupus, vasculitis, polyarthritis, sclerosing cholangitis, primary biliary cirrhosis and autoimmune hepatitis. Dairy products may also aggravate cysts and lumps in the thyroid and breasts, granulomatous diseases such as sarcoidosis and tuberculosis, and cancer of the lymphatic system such as lymphoma and leukaemia. I have found that in those with chronic or recurrent viral infections of the lymphatic system, such as glandular fever (Epstein Barr virus), it is necessary to eliminate all dairy products from the diet. These recommendations are based upon my own clinical experiences and not everyone will have had these same experiences, or indeed will agree with my recommendations. It is up to you to make up your own mind and if you have any of the above problems you may decide to follow the recipes and way of eating espoused in this book. The "proof of the pudding is in the eating," so why not try it for 4 to 6 months, although 12 months is better, and see if there is a change in your health?

Dairy products consist of animal milks and their derivatives, namely butter, cheese, cream, yoghurt, icecream and dairy chocolate.

Calcium Rich Foods

Food	Amount	Calcium (mg)
Fish (with the bones)		
Salmon (canned)	1 cup	431
Oysters, raw	1 cup	226
Sardines (with bones)	100gms(3.6oz)	300
Tuna (with bones)	100gms(3.6oz)	290
Fish (fresh, cooked)	100gms(3.6oz)	35
Legumes		
Tofu	112 gms(4oz)	80-150
Tempeh	112 gms(4oz)	172
Chickpeas	1 cup (cooked)	150
Tortillas, corn	2	120
Black beans	1 cup (cooked)	135
Soy milk (unfortified)	1 cup	60
Soy milk (fortified)	1 cup	300
Dairy		
Milk (cows)		
(whole)	1 cup	288
(skim)	1 cup	300
Goats milk	1 cup	295
Cheese (cheddar,Swiss)	42 gms(1.5oz)	300
Cottage cheese	1 cup	150
Feta cheese	28 gms(1oz)	129
Yoghurt	1 cup	294
Nuts and Seeds		
Brazil nuts	1 cup	260
Sunflower seeds (hulled)	1 cup	174
Sesame seeds (ground)	3 tablespoons	300
Almonds (hulled)	1 cup	300
Tahini (sesame paste)	1 tablespoon	85

Food	Amount	Calcium (mg)
Sea Vegetables (cooked)		
Wakame	1 cup	520
Agar-agar	1 cup	400
Kelp (kombu)	1 cup	305
Hijiki	1 cup	610
Dulse (dry)	1 cup	567
Green Vegetables (cooked)		
Parsley (raw)	1 cup	122
Bok choy	1 cup	200
Spinach	1 cup	178
Broccoli	1 cup	100
Beet greens	1 cup	165
Watercress (raw)	1 cup	53
Rhubarb	1 cup	348
Collard greens	1 cup	300
Dandelion greens	1 cup	147

As you can see, many different food groups contain calcium, such as green leafy vegetables, seeds, nuts and fish. One of the highest sources is sea vegetables (seaweeds) so popular in many Asian cultures, especially Japanese food. It is easy to get all the calcium you need without eating dairy products. All you need to do is have a varied and regular diet and if necessary take a calcium supplement.

Calcium Rich Herbal Vinegar for Salad Dressings

This is a nice one to make for yourself and your family. There are many herbs that are rich in bone building minerals including calcium. Herbs can be thought of as mineral-rich leafy vegetables. Try this little recipe to make yourself a mineral rich vinegar to use with your olive oil as a salad dressing.

Choose several of the following herbs:

Dandelion, Yellow dock, Red clover, Comfrey, Mugwort, Nettle and Plantain.

 Chop these fresh herbs to fill a one-litre jar. Add organic apple cider vinegar to herb mixture until jar is full. The vinegar will dissolve the minerals out of the herbs and keep them in solution, which makes them easily absorbed. Place a tight lid on the jar and leave in a cool dark place for 6 to 8 weeks.

After this time you may use it as a salad dressing, or dilute 1 tablespoon in 1 cup warm water and sip during meals You may sweeten this with blackstrap molasses which is also high in calcium.

Q.   Are these Recipes suitable for Children?

The recipes and principles found in this book are suitable for children, and indeed will help children with obesity, sluggish metabolism, recurrent infections, autoimmune diseases, chronic fatigue and allergies. I have found that it has helped a high percentage of children with common types of immune dysfunction such as asthma, sinus, hay fever and skin problems.

Children can be very fussy eaters, which makes it difficult to change their diet, however it does help if you do not keep unhealthy foods in the kitchen. If you find that it is necessary to keep your child on the principles of the Liver Cleansing Diet for more than 4 months, I suggest you give a calcium supplement of around 300 to 500 milligrams daily. Calcium is found in many other foods apart from dairy products. *See table on pages 61 to 62.*

Some very young children can suffer with severe liver disease and in some of these cases diet can play a very helpful role. In children with "Chronic Active Hepatitis" there is an autoimmune disease occurring, which makes the child allergic to their own liver. In this disease the principles found on *pages 20 to 27*, can make a huge difference to the outcome.

Another disease called "Galactosaemia" occurs when an enzyme needed to digest milk sugar is missing from the body, causing milk sugar to build up in the liver and other organs. This leads to liver scarring (cirrhosis), cataracts and brain damage, unless the baby is taken off milk and given a specific formula free of milk sugar.

The overuse of antibiotic drugs in children can damage the liver and that is why I am a firm believer in using natural methods to boost the immune system.

It is important to protect and support the liver function in children because their future environment will probably be more artificial and toxic than the present. Furthermore liver problems often first manifest at a relatively young age, and chronic liver diseases and cirrhosis still rank fourth as the leading disease-related cause of death for people aged between 25 and 44.

Q.   What if my Skin becomes too Yellow?

If you are consuming a large amount of yellow and orange coloured fruits and vegetables or their juices, you may find that your skin becomes a slightly yellow to orange colour. This is due to the high amount of the natural antioxidant carotenoid pigments present in these foods which gives you a natural bronze tinted "sun tanned" appearance. This is not dangerous in any way although this alarms some people. If this happens to you, simply reduce your consumption of orange coloured fruits and vegetables to a level that does not make you too yellow. If you take supplements of beta-carotene it is important to take only natural beta-carotene or a natural carotenoid complex.

Natural beta-carotene and its source foods are able to reduce the risk of many different types of cancer. Apart from beta-carotene, there are other important cancer preventing carotenoids found in brightly coloured fruits and vegetables such as alpha and gamma-carotene, lutein, and lycopene. Beta-carotene is a precursor to vitamin A and is converted to vitamin A in the liver. Vitamin A formed in this way is very good for the liver, and helps the liver to regulate cholesterol levels.

Just because vitamin A is good for the liver, it does not mean the more you take the better it will work. Indeed very high doses of vitamin A taken over long periods can be toxic to the liver and cause an elevation of liver enzymes. If you have been taking over 50,000 i.u. of vitamin A daily for over 6 months, you should reduce your intake or change to natural beta-carotene which is not liver toxic. Those with liver disease should not take more than 10,000i.u. of vitamin A on a daily basis. If you are taking cod liver oil for its many health advantages, it is important to check that your intake of vitamin A is not excessive because cod liver oil is high in vitamin A. Pregnant women should not take more than 5000 i.u. of vitamin A daily.

Q.   What if I have a Cyst in my Liver?

A cyst is the medical term used to describe a space of roundish or sac-like shape in some part of the body. It may be empty or contain watery or mucous types of fluid.

It is not uncommon to find one or several small cysts in the liver when a patient has an ultrasound scan or CAT scan of the abdomen for some reason. The vast majority of these cysts are found by chance as they do not produce any symptoms. These "simple cysts" usually arise because a small area of liver cells die or degenerate. The most common cause is advancing years and poor diet and lifestyle. Sometimes these cysts can be full of "fatty material" in those with a fatty liver. These cysts do not represent liver disease because the liver, being such a huge organ, has plenty of other areas containing healthy cells to enable liver function to remain normal.

If your doctor finds that you have one or several of these degenerative types of liver cysts (simple cysts), do not become alarmed. Obviously you do not want to develop many more of these cysts and thankfully it is easy to stop them from multiplying. In many cases it is possible to gradually shrink the cysts.

I recommend that you change your diet and follow the principles found in this book, and take an effective liver tonic. Those with simple liver cysts

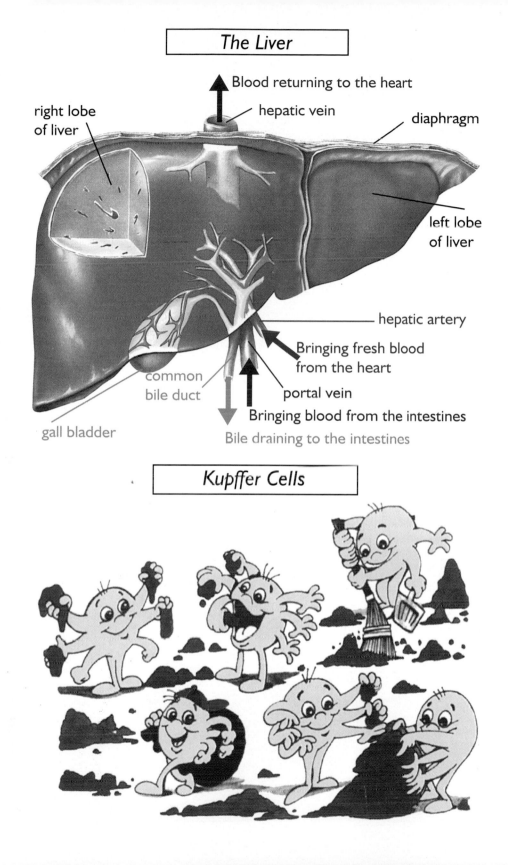

The Liver

Blood returning to the heart

right lobe of liver

hepatic vein

diaphragm

left lobe of liver

hepatic artery

Bringing fresh blood from the heart

common bile duct

portal vein

gall bladder

Bringing blood from the intestines

Bile draining to the intestines

Kupffer Cells

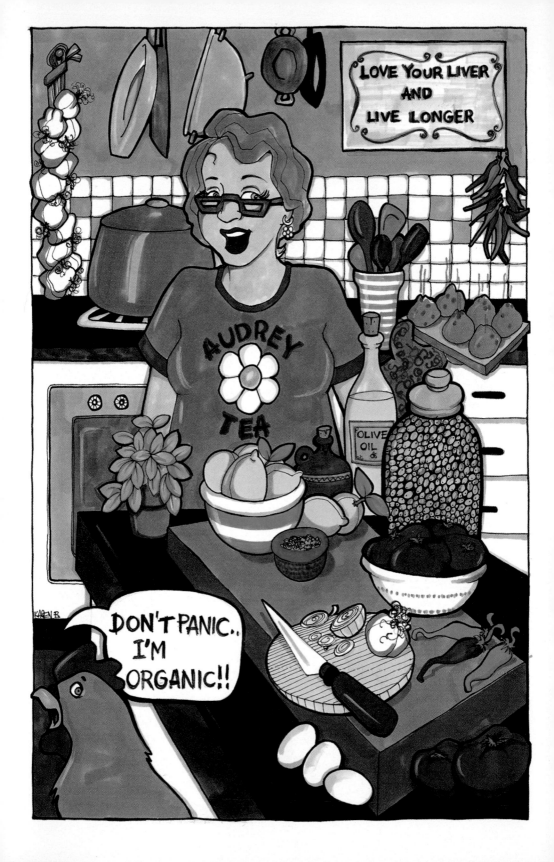

should avoid all dairy products, which is easy to do on the Liver Cleansing Diet. They should take vitamin E 1000 i.u. daily, Selenium 200 mcg daily, vitamin C 2000 mg daily, and boost their intake of essential fatty acids *(see page 20)*.

In areas where sheep and cattle raising are done, humans can become infected with the dog tapeworm Echinococcus granulosa, which can invade the liver causing cysts. These can be differentiated from simple cysts, which is important as they may require treatment to avoid rupture. Good standards of hygiene and regular worming of dogs can prevent these infections.

Q. Can I eat Liver on the Liver Cleansing Diet?

Some people not only love their liver, they love eating liver in their diet and are not sure if this is advantageous to their health. If you want to eat liver regularly I encourage you to find a reliable source of organically raised sheep and cattle so that their livers are not contaminated with growth hormones, antibiotics or pesticides. The animal's liver being the garbage disposal service of the body, will accumulate these toxins which will then end up in your liver.

Calf or lamb liver can be cooked in various ways that can be delicious and also provides a source of amino acids, vitamins A, E and B and iron. Well-respected Australian physician, Dr Ruth Cilento, discusses the health benefits of eating liver in her excellent book titled
"Heal Cancer", Hill of Content Publishing. On page 376 of this book she describes some tasty recipes containing calf and lambs liver.
Make sure that you wash the liver thoroughly and cook it well to remove any chemicals or microorganisms.

Q. What should I know if I have Gilbert's Syndrome?

I have included a question on Gilbert's syndrome because it is surprisingly common, affecting 2% to 5% of the population. Gilbert's Syndrome is an inherited disorder where there is a defect in the ability of the liver to excrete bile pigment (bilirubin).

This can lead to yellow skin and eye discolouration (jaundice), which fluctuates in degree. Gilbert's Syndrome is detected by finding a slightly raised bilirubin level in the blood with no other abnormalities of liver function and no signs of liver disease.

Gilbert's Syndrome is generally harmless and does not produce any symptoms, although some sufferers complain of excessive fatigue. Those with Gilbert's syndrome need only follow a healthy diet and avoid liver toxins such as excessive alcohol and liver toxic drugs. Bilirubin levels tend to rise if the diet is poor, and during fasting, or mild illnesses, which may cause the skin to yellow. Those with Gilbert's Syndrome should follow the principles of the Liver Cleansing Diet on *pages 20 to 27* and can be improved with a liver tonic *(see page 29)* designed to help the liver's detoxification pathways.

Gilbert's Syndrome does not require medical treatment or long term medical attention, and patients with this syndrome should not be led to believe that they have a liver disease. The major importance of establishing the correct diagnosis is so that the patient can be informed they do not have a serious disease, and unnecessary investigations can be avoided in the future.

Case Histories

In Hamilton, New Zealand, I met a young lady from New York who told me that she was on powerful drugs for auto-immune hepatitis and cirrhosis, which had developed two years before. The cortisone she had taken had given her a moon shaped face and many extra kilograms in body weight. She then changed to the drug Imuran, to avoid further weight gain. She had been told previously that she would be facing a liver transplant in the next ten years. I was most curious as to why a young woman would have such severe liver disease and I questioned her as to antecedent factors that could possibly be implicated in the aetiology of her disease. She had never suffered with viral hepatitis. She told me that her liver disease had followed a viral infection of the respiratory tract, and that many of her doctors had thought this to be the most likely cause. I was sceptical that this was truly the cause of her severe liver inflammation and cirrhosis, which takes much longer to develop, and must have been grumbling away for years. I then questioned her about her childhood and the answer became clear. She had been a sickly child, always suffering with ear infections and was always taking antibiotic drugs. Her parents had not understood that she needed to modify her diet to prevent these infections and had opted for the "safer" method of long-term and multiple antibiotic drugs. Unfortunately the excessive and often unnecessary use of antibiotics can cause liver damage, and also sensitise the immune system resulting in severe allergies and autoimmune diseases.

This young lady had achieved a great deal of improvement by following the principles of The Liver Cleansing Diet, but unfortunately she had already sustained chronic liver damage that was so severe it would be impossible to reverse it completely.

I have heard stories like this many times, and that is why I have included a small section on how to boost the immune system and overcome infections naturally with the aim of protecting the liver. *See page 50.*

George provides an interesting case history of how a few simple dietary changes can help men in midlife. He was a typical workaholic who ran a very busy company and had many outside interests that took all his time. Being a bachelor, he would eat on the run, usually popping into the local club and grabbing a meal of meat and overcooked vegetables followed by dessert. He grabbed a sandwich at lunchtime and snacked on bags of peanuts and chips and had the occasional glass of alcohol.

According to many he was not doing too badly and yet he was gradually putting on weight around the torso and was at least 20 kilograms (44 pounds) overweight. He also had several skin cancers that he was too busy to address.

One of his close friends told him about the principles of The Liver Cleansing Diet, and he gradually started to change as he was spending more time with this friend and found it easier to include raw fruits and vegetables in his diet. He also started taking some anti-oxidants, a liver tonic and selenium powder.

After six months of adopting these simple changes he had lost 42 pounds (19 kilograms) and had regained his youthful muscular physique. One morning he awoke with acute pain over the area of a large skin cancer on his wrist, which had become swollen and inflamed with what appeared to be an infection in the surrounding skin. He bathed the area with salt water and applied tea tree oil as an antiseptic.

Two weeks later the skin cancer shed itself off his wrist to leave an area of normal healthy skin. Over the next several months his other skin cancers became inflamed and shed themselves from his skin spontaneously.

This case history shows us how a few simple dietary changes to improve the function of the liver, can help both weight control and the immune system to become stronger.

In Fort Lauderdale, Florida

I met a woman aged in her late forties, who suffered with a severe case of fatty liver. She was carrying a lot of excess weight around her abdomen and had a roll of fat around the liver area. She complained of pains in the liver area and a bloated swollen abdomen. She had tried repeatedly to lose weight by following various low fat, low calorie diets, however she found them too difficult and too restrictive to maintain. Her doctor had done various tests, which showed that her liver was enlarged and swollen with fatty deposits, her gall bladder contained multiple small cholesterol stones, and her liver enzymes and cholesterol levels were elevated. The deposits of fat in the liver were so gross that some of them had formed sacs (cysts) full of thick yellow fat. It was these fatty cysts and possibly her gall stones that were causing her abdominal discomfort and bloating.

She was not a heavy drinker and her diet consisted of lots of processed foods and cheese. She was very worried about having a fatty liver and did not have a clue about how she could remove the fatty deposits from her liver. She was very relieved when she was able to talk to me at the end of my seminar, and indeed I always stay behind after the seminar to talk to anyone in the audience who needs special guidance. I explained to her that her liver was working opposite to how it was meant to work. Instead of burning fat it was storing fat.

First of all we would need to remove the excess fat from her liver before it could start to regulate fat metabolism efficiently. I started her on the liver cleansing program and prescribed a powerful liver tonic powder.

One year later I returned to Fort Lauderdale and met up with her again during a seminar. She looked much better having shed 27 kilograms (59 pounds), and no longer had a protuberant abdomen. She showed me her liver and gall bladder scan which showed that the liver was now of normal size and almost free of fatty deposits. The gallstones had gradually dissolved away and she had been able to avoid surgery, which would have been risky at her high weight. She related to me that initially it had been hard for her to change the types of foods she was eating, because the weight came off very slowly for the first six months and then started to come off rapidly. This change in the rate of weight loss only began when her liver scan showed that the fatty liver deposits had almost gone. It was at this point that her liver could start to burn fat from other areas of her body efficiently, as up until then the liver itself was being defatted. This is typical of people with a moderate to severe degree of fatty liver.

What can I do for my Pet's Liver?

Liver and bile problems are common in domestic animals such as dogs, cats and horses. The same factors that stress the human liver can adversely affect the function of the liver in your beloved pet or champion racehorse. Horse feed and pastures can contain pesticides, insecticides and unfriendly microorganisms, in which case the animal must be removed from the toxic agent immediately. Some chemicals used externally and internally to eradicate fleas can be liver toxins. Commercially produced pet food is often too high in damaged fats, salt and additives. Parasites and viruses can attack the animal liver, causing liver cysts and hepatitis. Many cases of obesity in cats and dogs are associated with a fatty liver. Horses can also suffer with a fatty liver.

Early diagnosis of liver disease in animals is important to prevent further destruction of the liver cells. The Health Advisory Service in Sydney has received many calls from distressed pet owners who have discovered on a blood test that their pet has abnormal liver function and elevated liver enzymes. In such cases nutritional medicine is often very effective and easy to implement.

Liver problems in Horses

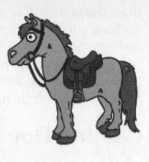

Liver problems in the horse may cause the animal to be depressed and sluggish, off its food and to lose weight. If ammonia levels build up in the blood stream the horse may display strange behaviour such as head pressing, wandering and yawning. Chlorophyll (the green pigment in the horses hay and chaff), combined with liver disease, can cause the unpigmented skin to become sensitive to sunlight (photosensitization). Skin irritation and inflammation result, and the horse should be protected from direct sunlight. There may be colour changes in the urine, faeces and eyes such as dark urine, pale faeces and yellowish membranes in the eyes and mouth.

Awareness and prompt attention to signs of possible liver dysfunction are essential for a good outcome.

Horses with disturbed liver function should have the following foods added to their regular feed:

Carrots, apples, ground linseed (flaxseed), ground sunflower seeds, fresh wheatgerm and oats. Supplements of cod liver oil can be mixed in the food along with a small amount of blackstrap molasses and Brewer's yeast.

If the horse has parasites such as worms, use raw garlic cloves, juiced, finely grated or crushed in a garlic press. The usual dose is 6 - 12 cloves daily mixed well throughout the food. You may be able to disguise the taste by mixing the garlic with black strap molasses. Anti-parasitic drugs may be required, however care should be taken not to use brands with liver toxic effects. Your vet may prescribe supplements of fat-soluble vitamins A, D, E, and K, as these may help the liver to repair itself.

If the horse has severe liver disease, the concentration of ammonia in the blood can be very high and a low protein diet will then be required. In this case alfalfa hay, soybean meal and other protein supplements should be avoided because their high protein content will further elevate blood ammonia levels. A grass hay based diet with a corn or oat concentrate is suitable, as it is low in protein and high in carbohydrates.

An animal version of the liver tonic powder called Livatone is available. It can easily be mixed into the horses feed. Generally 4 to 6 teaspoons of the powder twice daily is required, and in cases of liver inflammation or fatty liver, an extra 2 teaspoons twice daily can be added.

If the immune system is depressed and the horse has recurrent infections or inflammatory problems such as arthritis, or musculo-skeletal problems, there is a high chance that the animal lacks the vital mineral selenium. This can easily be supplemented in the form of a selenium yeast powder in a dose of 2 tablespoons daily, mixed well throughout the food. Selenium yeast powder is also beneficial in cases of infective or chronic hepatitis.

Cat and Dog Livers

Cats and Dogs with disturbed liver function can be helped with the following program:

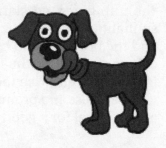

• Increase the amounts of cooked vegetables (eg.carrot, potato, pumpkin, beetroot, spinach, broccoli, and onions) in the diet. These vegetables can be steamed and then pureed in a blender, and mixed with some cooked wholegrain such as buckwheat, wheat, spelt, rice or barley. This can then be added to the meat or fish that the animal is receiving.
Oily fish such as tuna, sardines and salmon (expensive!) are excellent for the animal liver because of their high content of healing omega 3 essential fatty acids.

• Try to avoid fatty meats and remove skin and fat from the meat before cooking.

• Canned meat can be acceptable because food preparation time may not always be available, and you can add the cooked vegetables and grains to the canned meat or canned fish. Purchase brands of canned pet food that are promoting animal health by using low fat fresh ingredients in their products.

• Eggs are healthy for dogs and cats because they contain lecithin, along with the sulphur bearing amino acids to support the detoxification pathways in the liver. You may give the eggs raw, boiled or poached, and weekly allowances are 3 to 4 weekly for a medium sized dog, and 1 to 2 weekly for a medium sized cat. If your pet has a fatty liver, immune dysfunction or is overweight, avoid cows milk and all other dairy products. Lactose intolerance is not uncommon in dogs and cats and can cause bloating, gas and diarrhoea. It is easily overcome by eliminating cow's milk.

• Other liver healing foods for cats and dogs are ground linseed and sunflower seeds, fresh wheatgerm and Brewer's yeast powder. You can also use LSA (ground linseed, sunflower and almonds) which can be purchased pre-mixed, if you do not have the time to grind it freshly. Keep these things in the refrigerator or freezer away from the light.

If the animal has parasites such as worms (and most do), use raw garlic cloves either juiced, crushed in a garlic press or finely grated and mixed throughout the food at least three times a week. Your pet will not notice a problem with his or her social life!

If the animal has liver dysfunction or inflammation, an animal version of Livatone powder can be mixed into the food. This will also help those with fatty liver and obesity, making weight loss easier.

The dosage is:

For dogs -   Small size   1 teaspoon daily
                  Medium size   1+1/2 teaspoons daily
                  Large size   2 teaspoons daily
For cats -
                  Small to medium size   1/2 teaspoon daily
                  Large size   1 teaspoon daily

NOTE:
Cats a very susceptible to liver damage from the analgesic drug paracetamol. Even one tablet of paracetamol can cause fatal liver failure in cats.

The most glamorous case history of how the liver can affect an animal is reflected in the story of "Kala Beat," named " Horse of the Year" in 1995 by the Northern Rivers Racing Association, for its racing wins in Northern NSW. This great champion started to lose his energy and stopped winning races that should have been a snack for him. The veterinarian discovered that the horse had an elevated liver enzyme count, with a reading of 90, instead of the normal below 30 that is found in horses. The owners had heard of the good results being achieved by people taking the liver tonic Livatone, and they commenced Kala Beat on the Livatone in horse sized doses after contacting the Health Advisory Service.

After 10 weeks of the Livatone treatment the horse's liver enzyme levels were down to 33, which was much better than the horse had maintained in several years. The owners were delighted and recommended Kala Beat on the racing circuit with fabulous wins ensuing. Unfortunately they forgot to tell the team at the Health Advisory Service, who would have bet on this liver happy champion had only they known!

Liver Diseases

Liver Tumours

A liver tumour is an abnormal growth or mass found in the liver.

Secondary Tumours

The most common liver tumour is a secondary (metastatic) tumour. This means that the tumour has spread to the liver (metastasised) from its original source of origin. The most common sources of origin are cancers of the intestines, breast or bronchial tubes (lungs). The tumour will take root in the liver and continue to grow, eventually causing liver enlargement and perhaps yellow jaundice.

Primary Tumours

Primary tumours begin their existence in the liver. Tumours that originate in the liver may be benign or malignant. The most common are malignant. Diagnosis is made with imaging techniques such as ultrasound scan, CAT scan or MRI of the liver.

A. Primary Liver Cancer

Primary liver cancer refers to cancer cells originating in the liver. Primary cancer of the liver is one of the most common cancers worldwide, although much less common in the Western Hemisphere. It usually presents itself in persons below the age of 50 years.

The symptoms usually progress rapidly and consist of weight loss, loss of appetite, fever, abdominal pain and swelling. The liver feels enlarged and irregular. Primary liver cancer does not have a good outlook, and this is why it is important to avoid the factors that cause it. Early diagnosis and correction of these factors can prevent primary liver cancer.

Factors that increase the risk of liver cancer are:

Chronic infection with hepatitis B and C viruses. *See page 77*

Haemochromatosis . *See page 84*

Alcoholism

Possible association may exist with long term ingestion of high oestrogen doses (sometimes seen in transvestites) and androgenic steroids.

B. Benign Liver Tumours

Benign (non-cancerous) liver tumours may grow in the liver and the most common types are called a haemangioma and an adenoma.

Haemangiomas consist of a tangle of dilated blood vessels somewhere in the liver. The tumour is often found incidentally because it does not usually cause any symptoms. Haemangiomas do not require treatment, although rough sports should be avoided if the tumour is large because of the remote possibility of rupture.

Adenomas are associated with use of the oral contraceptive pill or high dose hormone replacement therapy, and they usually regress after the hormones are discontinued. Those on the oral contraceptive pill and/or hormone tablets should have their liver function checked annually. These benign tumours are easily seen on an ultra sound scan of the liver. They do not develop into cancer.

Cirrhosis

This is the term used to describe the end stages of liver disease where chronic inflammation of liver cells has caused an extensive build up of scar tissue in the liver. Scar tissue is the same as collagen as it is tough fibrous tissue, which replaces damaged liver cells. This scar tissue is not functional and cannot do the work of liver cells. Liver cells known as stellate cells produce the scar tissue to protect themselves from the inflammation that is occurring in the liver. This inflammation is produced by free radicals generated by viruses, toxins, unhealthy fats, alcohol, and some drugs or antibodies that are attacking liver cells. A healthy liver does not have many stellate cells and they do not produce excessive amounts of scar tissue. In contrast, in a liver that is chronically inflamed, the stellate cells become activated and they multiply and produce excessive collagen.

A cirrhotic liver is hardened with scar tissue, which reduces its blood supply. There is not enough healthy liver tissue to perform the metabolic and detoxification processes that the liver must perform to keep the body healthy.

Cirrhosis of the liver is the fourth most common cause of death among people aged between 30 and 50. Chronic hepatitis (caused by the hepatitis B and C virus) is gaining on alcohol as the leading cause of cirrhosis.

With millions of people worldwide suffering with cirrhosis, it is impractical to rely exclusively on expensive and in short supply, liver transplants as the ultimate cure.

Causes of cirrhosis are:

Excessive alcohol, chronic hepatitis B and C infection, immune liver diseases such as auto-immune hepatitis and primary biliary cirrhosis, metabolic disorders such as Wilson's disease and Haemochromatosis, adverse reactions to some drugs such as methotrexate and vascular disorders of the liver.

Signs of advanced cirrhosis may include:

Spider naevi - spider shaped capillaries on the skin
Excessive bruising
Jaundice (yellow discolouration of skin and eyes)
Altered liver size
Enlarged spleen
Clubbing of the ends of the fingers
Ascites (fluid build up in the abdomen)
Swelling of the limbs with fluid (oedema)
A flapping tremor of the hands
Mental confusion and disorientation

To prevent and reduce cirrhosis from various causes it is necessary to do several things:

• Increase antioxidants, which neutralise free radicals.

These are natural vitamin E 1000 i.u. daily (some people may need 2000 i.u.), vitamin C 1000 mg three times daily and selenium 200 mcg daily.

Vitamin E is able to reduce the ability of the stellate cells to manufacture collagen and so reduces scar tissue production. Vitamin E can also soften existing scar tissue and therefore improve blood flow to the liver, which is essential for regeneration of the liver cells. Vitamin E assists in the maintenance of high levels of glutathione, which is the most powerful liver antioxidant to prevent cirrhosis. A clinical study of hepatitis C sufferers not responding to interferon therapy, showed that nearly 50% improved dramatically with 800 i.u. daily of vitamin E. These are the reasons why a high dose of vitamin E is required. Use only natural vitamin E which is known as d-alpha tocopherol.

Natural beta-carotene is another antioxidant that is able to improve liver function, and can be taken as part of a liver tonic or by itself and doses range from 5000 to 15000 i.u. daily. It is vital to also obtain plenty of beta-carotene and its related carotenoids from eating a wide variety of raw brightly coloured fruits and vegetables. Beta-carotene is converted in the body to vitamin A. Beta-carotene, other carotenoids and vitamin A exert a vital anti-cancer effect in those with cirrhosis. This will reduce the risk of cirrhotic livers developing cancer. Those with liver disease need to be careful not to take excessive amounts of vitamin A *(see page 64)* and should not take more than 10,000 i.u. daily.

• Take a liver tonic that contains the essential nutrients to support the liver's ability to break down and excrete toxins *(see page 29)*. This will reduce the damage that toxins can inflict upon liver cells. For cirrhosis, I would recommend a liver tonic in powder form in a dose of 1 teaspoon twice daily in raw juices.

• Many people with cirrhosis have a problem with bruising or excessive bleeding because the liver does not manufacture sufficient clotting factors. This can be helped by the daily consumption of a fresh juice made with a mixture of raw dark green leafy vegetables. Good vegetables to use for this purpose are spinach, kale, beetroot tops, parsley, mint, watercress, wheatgrass and alfalfa sprouts which are high in vitamin K. Vitamin K will help to reduce this deficiency of clotting factors and will reduce bruising and bleeding. For some juice recipes *see page 168.*

• Minimise the use of all medications, especially liver toxins such as alcohol, analgesic drugs (especially paracetamol and narcotics), anti-inflammatory drugs and antibiotics. Avoid using household and workplace chemicals such as insecticides, pesticides, chlorine, bleach, paints, glues and solvents.

• Obtain your protein by combining grains, raw nuts, raw seeds, sprouts and legumes. The cirrhotic liver cannot handle large amounts of concentrated protein and for this reason minimise, or even better, avoid the consumption of red meat and poultry. If you eat too much animal protein ammonia levels will build up in the blood stream causing mental fatigue and confusion. The principles of the Liver Cleansing Diet found on *pages 20 to 27* are a good guideline to follow. If your liver function is very poor you will have to avoid the recipes in this book that contain meat and poultry. You may have to avoid all animal protein (including eggs, seafood, red meats, white meats, and dairy products), and confine your protein sources to legumes (beans, peas, lentils), grains, cereals, seeds, sprouts and nuts. In this situation you will need to take supplemental Taurine 1000mg twice daily, and vitamin B 12 100 mcg daily. Small doses of the amino acids glutamine, cysteine, and glycine can be taken in the form of a liver tonic to increase glutathione levels. Glutathione and glutamine improve leaky bowel syndrome and this helps to reduce absorption of toxic ammonia from the bowel. Large doses of amino acids should be avoided in those with end stage cirrhosis and liver failure. Make sure that you remain under the supervision of your specialist and a good dietician.

• Avoid constipation by consuming plenty of raw fruits and vegetables, and grind fresh seeds (flaxseed, pumpkinseed, sunflower seeds etc) and almonds, and mix with oat bran to increase intestinal fibre. This fibre will speed the passage of toxins out of the bowels and reduce the ability of these toxins to recirculate back to the liver.

• Drink at least two litres (4 pints) of water daily to increase excretion of toxins through the kidneys. This will reduce the workload of the compromised cirrhotic liver.

• If the bowel function is poor because of constipation and excess populations of unhealthy bacteria, this can lead to excessive fermentation of the bowel contents, which will increase absorption of toxic ammonia and other nitrogen compounds from the bowel. A healthy liver can convert nitrogen into urea, which is excreted in the urine. In patients with end stage cirrhosis and very poor liver function, the liver is not able to handle these high levels of ammonia and toxic brain symptoms may occur. In this situation bowel function should be improved by increasing raw food fibre and taking supplements of the healthy lactobacillus bacteria. Enemas and colonic irrigations can also help if there is severe constipation and auto-intoxication from the bowel.

• Fifty percent of your diet should consist of raw vegetables and fruits. Dressings can be made with organic vinegars (balsamic, apple cider vinegar etc) and cold pressed vegetable oils. Drink one or two glasses of raw vegetable juices daily. Replace regular coffee with dandelion or cereal coffees.

• Eat cruciferous vegetables, garlic and onions to help the detoxification ability of the liver.

• Make sure that you are not consuming excessive iron and that your body's total iron content is within normal limits. This can be confirmed with a simple blood test known as "iron studies". Post menopausal women and men may have an excess of iron, which even if slight, can increase liver damage. Hepatitis viruses thrive in high-iron environments and surplus iron can cause immune dysfunction.

Reducing iron intake can increase the success rate of interferon therapy. Avoid iron-enriched cereals, vitamin pills containing iron, liver, red meats, and molasses and cooking in iron pots.

• Take lecithin in the form of granules (must be fresh and refrigerated) with your cereal in a dose of 2 to 3 tablespoons daily. Lecithin can also be taken as part of a liver tonic and in capsule form. Lecithin will increase choline levels in the liver. Choline increases the liver enzyme called "collagenase" which is very effective in breaking down collagen (scar tissue), which prevents and reduces cirrhosis. Lecithin has been proven in controlled animal studies to prevent alcoholic induced cirrhosis. Trials are now being done in humans to try and reproduce these exciting effects.

• Alpha-lipoic acid 300mg to 600mg daily.

Other nutritional therapies that are still being studied and show promise are

S - adenosyl - L - methionine and N-acetyl cysteine (NAC) which help to maintain levels of the liver antioxidant glutathione. The progress of these therapies can be followed on the Internet and in future medical journals. **Ref 4 and 5.**

The active principle of liquorice root is called glycyrrhizin, and has been used in Japan for many years to treat liver diseases including cirrhosis. It has been used as an injection, and controlled trials have shown that it can produce an improvement in liver enzymes and liver biopsies. **Ref 6.** It is not known if oral preparations of liquorice root would have this beneficial effect. Large quantities of liquorice root can cause high blood pressure so only a qualified herbalist should prescribe it.

Hepatitis

Hepatitis is a general term used to describe inflammation of the liver. This means that there are too many inflammatory chemicals being produced and released in the liver which damages the liver cells (hepatocytes). Your doctor will be able to diagnose hepatitis, even of a mild degree, by doing a blood test to check the level of liver enzymes *(see page 98)* If the liver enzymes are elevated this means you have some degree of liver inflammation occurring.

What causes Hepatitis?

It can be caused by excessive alcohol, toxic chemicals, incorrect diet, some drugs, autoimmune diseases, some diseases of the biliary system and viral infections. Viruses, which attack liver cells, are known as hepatitis A, B, C,

D, E, F and G. Other viruses of both new and old varieties can also attack the liver such as Epstein Barr virus (glandular fever virus) and the cocksackie virus.

Hepatitis A

Hepatitis A is also known as infectious hepatitis. It is easily spread through food or liquids, cutlery, bed linen and skin exposed to faeces contaminated with the virus. Transmission can be avoided by adopting high standards of personal hygiene especially in the preparation of food. International travellers are at risk of catching hepatitis A and should consider preventative vaccination. While travelling, drink only boiled or bottled carbonated water, avoid eating all raw fish and shellfish, and use disinfectant soaps for the hands.

The virus attacks the liver producing an acute illness with symptoms of nausea, loss of appetite, vomiting, fatigue and jaundice. This illness usually lasts for several weeks and resolves quickly once the virus is cleared from the body. In those who are run down to start with there may be a prolonged or relapsing illness and this occurs in around 15% of cases. However unlike hepatitis B or C, a chronic illness does not develop from the hepatitis A virus, and once the virus is cleared from the body a permanent immunity is acquired. The hepatitis A virus does not cause cirrhosis.

There is now a vaccine, which is highly effective in preventing hepatitis A. In those recently exposed to hepatitis A, an injection of gamma globulin can reduce the risk of infection if given within 24 hours of exposure.

Hepatitis C - an Epidemic Problem

Infection with the hepatitis C virus is common, and there are around 300 million people worldwide who have contracted this virus.

Hepatitis C virus (HCV) is classed as the fastest-growing infectious disease in Australia and America, and this upward trend is set to continue. If it does, by the year 2010 we can expect many thousands of people to have developed HCV- related cirrhosis, with many requiring liver transplants.

Researchers estimate that in Australia, 0.5 to 1% of the general population tests positive to hepatitis C virus. In the USA the incidence is estimated to be around 1.8% of the population, while in many parts of Asia infection rates are much higher than this.

HCV was only identified in 1988. Previously it was known as non-A, non-B hepatitis. HCV is 10 times more infectious than HIV (the AIDS virus), and unpublished research in Victoria suggests it may survive for long periods on needles and other equipment.

In the 1980's, AIDS was the major public health challenge for community based doctors. Now in the late 1990's and during the turn of the next millennium, hepatitis C has this dubious honour.

Do you need a test for Hepatitis C?

If you received a blood transfusion or blood products before routine screening of donor blood was introduced (before February 1990), or if you have ever shared equipment (needles, spoons, swabs, tourniquets, etc) for injecting any drugs, it is important that you ask your doctor for a blood test to check for hepatitis C. If you have been tattooed, had body piercing or needle-stick injuries, you should also consider being tested for hepatitis C.

How can you catch the Hepatitis C virus?

The virus is nearly always transmitted via blood to blood contact.

This occurs through the sharing of equipment to inject drugs, needle-stick injuries in health care workers, and unsafe techniques of body piercing and tattooing.

Cocaine snorting is recognised increasingly as a potential mode of transmission through the sharing of contaminated straws.

It is possible that the virus may be transmitted to a baby from an infected mother, although this occurs in only around 6% of such cases. Infection of the baby through breast-feeding from an infected mother is very uncommon, however great care should be taken to avoid nipple trauma.

Razor blades and toothbrushes can become contaminated with blood, so it is important not to share these things. Always wear gloves when wiping up blood spills, using paper towels and good quality bleach.

Nowadays the risk of catching hepatitis C from a blood transfusion is extremely low, because blood banks now screen all donated blood.

Sexual transmission of the virus is very unlikely, although it is important to practice safe sexual techniques to avoid blood to blood contact. The risk of sexual transmission is estimated to be around 4%.

Initial Effects of Infection with Hepatitis C Virus

People are generally completely unaware that they have contracted this virus because it does not produce any symptoms in the early or acute stages of the infection. During the first 3 to 6 months after infection, the virus replicates itself rapidly and the immune system tries to fight it by producing antibodies against it.

Unfortunately in 80 to 85 percent of infected people, the virus is not eliminated and becomes a long-term inhabitant of the body. In other words, the infection becomes chronic. In a significant percentage of people with chronic infection, there are no signs or symptoms of disease and many are unaware that they are carrying an infection that can be transmitted to others through contact with their blood.

Long Term Effects of the Hepatitis C Virus.

The amount of long term liver damage caused by the hepatitis C virus varies from person to person, and those with a strong immune system and a healthy diet and lifestyle will have a much better outcome.

In those who become infected with this virus we find the following approximate outcomes:

15 to 20 percent of people will completely eliminate the virus from their bodies within 3 to 6 months (much like we overcome the flu virus).
60 percent of people will develop a long-term (chronic) infection that may not cause any problems or may go on to varying degrees of liver damage.
20 to 25 percent of people will suffer serious liver damage, although this takes around 20 years to develop. In this group, 10 to 15 percent will remain stable and be able to survive with their disease, while 10 percent will go on to develop liver failure and/or liver cancer. Chronic infection may also cause severe loss of liver cells and extensive scarring of the liver which is called cirrhosis.
The death rate from chronic hepatitis C infection is around 5 to 10% and is due to end stage liver failure or the development of liver cancer.

Hepatitis B

This is a common viral infection of the liver and worldwide there are estimated to be over 300 million carriers.

How is Hepatitis B spread?

The hepatitis B virus can be transmitted between humans by blood or sexual secretions. Good hygiene is imperative in reducing the spread of this virus because it can enter the body in many ways- through sexual contact, sores and cuts in the skin, body contact sports, sharing infected needles, razor blades and toothbrushes. Do not share these items, wash your hands regularly with hot water and soap, and cover open wounds in the skin. Hepatitis B virus can also be transmitted where improperly sterilised equipment is used for tattooing, ear piercing and acupuncture. The hepatitis B virus can survive outside the body for long periods of time.

It is one of the most common sexually transmitted diseases in the world. The use of condoms with new sexual partners will protect you.

General social contact in the work place and society will not spread the hepatitis B virus. It is not generally spread by food, sweat, tears, coughing, sneezing or kissing. The virus is killed by disinfectants (including bleach) and boiling water, which is why good hygiene is so important in the prevention of this infection.

You may become infected from a carrier of the virus who does not know that they have the virus in their body because often it does not produce any symptoms of illness.

All blood donors are screened for hepatitis B and C viruses.

What are the symptoms of Hepatits B infection?

After initial contact with the virus symptoms take on average, around 60 to 90 days to develop. Adults will develop symptoms that vary in severity from mild to severe, and include yellow discolouration of the skin and eyes (jaundice), loss of appetite and nausea, abdominal pains, fatigue, fever, and joint pains. Although these unpleasant symptoms may last for many weeks to months, recovery without any long-term effects is the usual outcome. Those who make a recovery have a good immune system, which eradicates the virus for life.

In a small percentage of people the virus remains in the body long-term and is infectious to others. These people are known as carriers. This chronic form of hepatitis B may silently damage your liver as the years go by, and a significant percentage of chronic carriers will develop liver cancer or cirrhosis. This is particularly so if the carrier has a poor diet and unhealthy lifestyle which compromises the immune system. Those carriers who are positive for the "e antigen" of hepatitis B are more likely to develop liver disease.

Infants infected by their mothers at birth may not suffer a serious illness initially, however they have the highest risk of becoming long-term carriers.

Prevention

Since 1983 a vaccine against hepatitis B has been available. This vaccine is made using techniques of genetic engineering. Vaccination is a good idea for those who are at a high risk of catching hepatitis B.

High risk people are health care workers, haemodialysis patients, low socioeconomic groups, homosexual men, injection drug users, prostitutes, the sexually promiscuous, infants and children of immigrants from disease-endemic areas, infants born to infected mothers, sexual and household contacts of infected persons. Because hepatitis B is such a widespread infection it is recommended that children be routinely vaccinated against this virus.

A hepatitis B immunoglobulin injection is also available to reduce the risk of infection in those people who know they may have just contacted the virus (after needle stick injury or contamination with infected blood etc.) This immunoglobulin injection should be given as soon as possible (within 24 hours) after the exposure.

How can you reduce liver damage from Hepatitis Viruses ?

Medical Treatment

Treatment is based on the drug Interferon-alpha (IFN-alpha). This drug is given by injection and a common dosage regime is 3 million units, three times a week, for 12 months.

The majority of patients who will ultimately respond to IFN tend to do so within the first 3 months of treatment. If there is no real improvement after this time the drug is generally stopped. Interferon often causes a wide range of side effects such as a "flu like illness," suppression of the bone marrow, infections, mood changes and immune dysfunction.

Trials of therapy using a combination of the drugs IFN and Ribavirin are showing some good results. Much more research is being done into specific antiviral drugs such as NS3 proteinase and effective vaccines. Large amounts of money are needed to maintain this ongoing research which is essential in the face of this rapidly spreading epidemic.

The aim of Interferon treatment is to eliminate hepatitis C virus infection and prevent liver damage and liver cancer. Interferon alone eliminates the virus in only 10 to 20% of patients. Another 25 to 40% respond but subsequently relapse. These patients may achieve much better results with Interferon/Ribavirin combination therapy. In many cases it is impossible to eradicate the hepatitis C virus from the body and patients find it difficult to tolerate drug side effects.

It is therefore not surprising that sufferers are turning towards nutritional and herbal therapies to fight the virus. Natural therapies will not usually be able to eradicate the virus from the body, however they will definitely help to prevent the virus from damaging the liver. This approach is very successful and can keep the virus in a dormant or harmless state so that it does not damage liver cells.

To achieve this we must help the immune system by doing the following:

- Follow the principles of the Liver Cleansing Diet found on *pages 20 to 27*, which gives comprehensive and easy to follow strategies to use everyday to repair and rejuvenate the liver.
- It is vital to eat foods rich in natural sulphur containing compounds such as onions, garlic, free range eggs and cruciferous vegetables (broccoli, Brussels sprouts, cauliflower and cabbage).
- Drink raw fresh vegetable and fruit juices made daily with a juice-

extracting machine.

• Increase consumption of essential fatty acids found in foods such as freshly ground flaxseed, avocados, raw nuts and seeds, cold pressed vegetable and seed oils and oily fish such as salmon, sardines and tuna. Essential fatty acids will repair the membranes surrounding the liver cells and reduce inflammation. Capsules of evening primrose oil, flaxseed oil, lecithin and blackcurrant seed oil can also be taken daily to boost healing essential fatty acids.

• A liver tonic is vital to support the detoxification pathways in the liver, thereby helping the liver to break down toxic chemicals. A well-designed liver tonic is able to repair liver damage and renew the growth of new and healthy liver cells. It will also support the filter inside the liver, which removes microorganisms, dead cells and toxins from the blood stream. This will keep your blood stream clean and free of dangerous toxins and microorganisms. You will require a powerful multi-action synergistic natural liver formula that is able to support all aspects of liver function. For more information on the ingredients that should be combined in an effective liver tonic *see page 29*. Such a tonic is a natural dietary supplement free of chemicals and drugs and is very safe to take on a long-term basis. It is easy to take in capsule and/or powder form and should be taken in a dose of 2 capsules twice daily, or one teaspoon twice daily stirred into juice. Take just before meals. Its regular use not only repairs and heals liver cells, it also supports the fat burning function of the liver which helps to keep weight under control, reduce blood cholesterol and triglyceride levels and promotes healthy bile and gall bladder function.

• Selenium Designer Yeast Powder is a natural dietary supplement that can help all those with a viral infection of the liver, liver inflammation or a weakened immune system. It is also helpful for those with auto-immune diseases.

The mineral selenium will support the immune system and reduce the ability of the liver viruses to replicate. This is vitally important because the amount of liver damage caused by the hepatitis viruses is related to the ability of the viruses to multiply inside the liver cells.

It has been categorically proven that patients who are deficient in trace minerals such as selenium and zinc will have more severe viral infections resulting in more severe tissue damage. Ref 2.

Selenium has been called the "viral birth control pill' as it reduces viral replication. Selenium yeast powders are an excellent and highly bio-available form of selenium combined with its synergistic cofactors such as zinc, boron, molybdenum, manganese, anti-oxidants and amino acids. These minerals are helpful for viral infections of the liver, chronic systemic viral infections, a weakened immune system and inflammatory diseases. They are able to strengthen the immune system, which will help to keep viruses in a dormant and harmless state.

Dosage of powder is two teaspoons daily stirred into fresh fruit or vegetable juices. Patients who are taking selenium yeast powders will notice a big improvement in energy levels and find that after several months the appearance of their hair and skin will improve. For those who do not like powders, Vitaglow Selemite B tablets can be used as an alternative.

• Vitamin C should be taken in a dose of 1000 mg three times daily, to reduce viral replication and inflammation. Vitamin C is the most important vitamin for the liver and reduces liver damage inflicted by viruses and toxic chemicals. Good sources of vitamin C are citrus fruits, kiwi fruits, strawberries and red and green capsicums. Organically grown produce is best to reduce exposure of the liver to pesticides and insecticides.

• Olive Leaf Extract can be taken in a dose of 500 to 1000mg three times daily just before meals. Use a capsule containing at least a 10% extract of the active ingredient, which is called "oleuropein."

Extensive research has shown that Olive Leaf Extract can reduce replication of most viruses and indeed is an effective and non-toxic natural anti-biotic. **Ref 10**.

• Alpha-lipoic acid 300mg to 600mg daily is a powerful antioxidant

In Summary

Excellent results have been achieved by using nutritional programs in many patients with chronic viral infections of the liver. This can also reduce damage caused by any long-term systemic viral infection, including the AIDS virus.

The most important strategy is to begin such a program as early as possible and to stay on it long-term. It is possible to restore normal liver function in many chronic viral hepatitis sufferers provided they also stick to a healthy diet and drug free life-style.

At the very least a significant improvement in liver function and well being will always be achieved, provided you do not wait until end-stage liver disease has set in.

Haemochromatosis

The genetic disorder of Haemochromatosis or iron overload, is the opposite to iron deficiency. Many people believe that the body has a high requirement for dietary iron and think the more they eat the better their health will be. This is not so for everyone and is a very individual thing. Indeed the disease of iron overload is all too common and unfortunately remains grossly under diagnosed.

Haemochromatosis affects those of Celtic, Anglo and Nordic origins and is most common in those of strong Irish descent. It affects as many as 1 in 200 Caucasians. It is now considered to be the most common genetic disorder and close to 24 million people worldwide may be at risk of this severe disease.

Haemochromatosis is a silent killer and creeps up on unwitting sufferers causing severe organ damage. This damage is easily prevented and treated by the equivalent of the old fashioned leech treatment-draining of blood, provided it is detected early enough.

It is detected easily and inexpensively with a simple blood test called "serum iron studies". It is so easy to diagnose that some have dubbed this disease "a diagnosis waiting to be made".

An average person has around one gram of iron in their body, whereas a sufferer of Haemochromatosis can store around twenty grams, enough to set off airport metal detectors in severe cases!

The reason it is often not detected until permanent damage has already occurred, is because it may not produce any early symptoms, and when it does, the symptoms may be vague and diverse and attributed to other causes. For example, when the disease is at its most treatable, sufferers are often teenagers, or in their 20's and 30's, and complain of fatigue, abdominal discomfort and aches and pains. These things may be mistaken for Chronic Fatigue Syndrome or viral illness. If the disease progresses undiagnosed, toxic iron levels will build up in the liver, pancreas, heart, skin and joints leading to severe damage in these organs. In the late stages of untreated Haemochromatosis a sufferer has a 200-fold higher risk of liver cancer than a normal person does and the only option is a liver transplant.

Treatment

Eating foods high in iron may worsen the disease but will not cause it, as the problem is a genetic disorder of iron metabolism. Indeed, iron is so widespread in foods that it is virtually impossible to avoid it and by trying to do this, you could develop nutritional deficiencies. However, sufferers would be wise to avoid a regular intake of red meats and organ meats. Patients can enjoy a normal and varied diet, along the principles of the Liver Cleansing Diet, provided they have their blood removed regularly. They must be monitored with regular blood tests under the supervision of a specialist (haematologist).

One gentleman who suffered with liver damage caused by Haemochromatosis called the Health Advisory Service to ask dietary questions. He had stopped all green leafy vegetables such as broccoli and spinach because they contain iron. This is not a good idea because these types of vegetables are very important for healthy liver function and help to heal and repair liver damage. Provided regular venesection (blood letting) is done, the excess iron in the blood can be removed efficiently. Restricting the intake of fresh raw vegetables is not a good idea and will result in nutritional deficiencies and impaired liver function.

Taking iron supplements can be very harmful in this disorder and it is important to check your blood levels of iron before committing to long term supplementation with iron tablets.

Treatment is life saving and consists of the regular removal of venous blood which is called venesection. Normal health and life expectancy can be achieved if the excess iron can be removed through regular venesection before organ damage has occurred.

It is a good idea to take supplemental Vitamin E 1000 to 2000 i.u. daily, and selenium 200 mcg daily, to reduce free radical damage caused by excess iron. If there is liver damage, a natural liver tonic can help, but make sure that it does not contain any iron.

I enclose a letter from a gentleman in Victoria, Australia

Dear Health Advisory Service
Since my original contact as a Haemochromatosis sufferer I am now a member of the Haemochromatosis Society of Australia Support Group. I am very motivated to promote awareness and early detection of this disease. Haemochromatosis is manageable when detected early but usually by the time symptoms become evident, severe organ damage has already occurred. With 1 in 10 of the population being a carrier, and 1 in every 200 to 300 being a sufferer, a significant percentage of the population are at risk. For example with a population of 80,000 in Ballarat City, and a regional population above 100,000, there is the probability of over 300 cases of Haemochromatosis within reach. Unfortunately, statistics have shown that only 10% of cases have been detected. The chance to alert and detect these cases before serious damage sets in, is a very attractive course to follow. If you are able to raise awareness in your area of influence, and lead even one sufferer to an earlier diagnosis, then very good works will have been achieved.

For more information contact:
Haemochromatosis Information Service.
412 Musgrave Rd, Coopers Plains QLD. 4108.
Phone:
Australian callers - 07-3345 7583
International callers - 617-3345 7583
Web sites:
http://www.emi.net/~iron_iod/ *or*
http://home.istar.ca/~chcts/index.htm

Wilson's Disease

This is a very rare inherited disorder causing an inability of the body to metabolise the mineral copper. It results is very high and toxic levels of copper building up in the liver and parts of the brain, leading to liver scarring (cirrhosis) and neurological disease. Children affected with Wilson's disease develop liver problems, whereas young adults have more neurological problems, such as movement and speech disorders and eventually dementia. Diagnosis and treatment of this severe disease is performed by a specialist and involves the use of drugs such as D-penicillamine, triethylene tetramine and/or zinc supplements. Effective treatment depends upon early diagnosis before permanent damage has set in. Wilson's disease is one of the few inherited metabolic disorders for which there is effective treatment.

Nutritional medicine can help patients with Wilson's disease and consists of:

Avoidance of foods high in copper eg. organ meats, liver, shellfish, nuts, legumes, whole grains and their cereals and chocolates.

Eat plenty of cruciferous vegetables, garlic, onions and ginger.

Eat small regular meals.

Ensure a high fluid intake of 2 litres daily to reduce kidney stones.

Vitamin B 6 and multi-mineral tablets (without copper) must be taken to reduce the side effects of D-penicillamine. The multi-mineral tablet should contain the mineral molybdenum (30 mcg to 5mg daily may be required)

Zinc chelate 600 mg per day increases the excretion of copper.

Anti-oxidants such as vitamin C 2000 to 3000 mg daily, vitamin E 2000 i.u. daily and selenium 200 mcg daily will reduce free radical damage caused by the excessive copper.

Sclerosing Cholangitis

This is an inflammatory disease of the bile ducts, which eventually become scarred and narrowed ducts (tubes). It is thought to be autoimmune in origin, which means that the immune system produces antibodies, which attack the bile ducts in the liver. This is supported by the fact that 50% of patients with sclerosing cholangitis have inflammatory disease of the bowel.

There may be no definite symptoms, except for general fatigue and it may be picked up in a blood test by finding a high level of the liver enzyme alkaline phosphatase. In more severe cases, symptoms such as itching skin (pruritus), abdominal pain and yellow discolouration of skin and eyes (jaundice) may occur. The veins in the liver may become blocked by scar tissue, which causes an increase in the venous pressure in the liver. This is called portal hypertension. A biopsy (tissue sample) of the liver confirms the diagnosis of sclerosing cholangitis.

The outcome is variable with 50% of patients being able to have a reasonably normal life over many years. Strong anti-inflammatory drugs are sometimes helpful, but not without side effects. Those who do poorly will require a liver transplant.

Sclerosing cholangitis can respond very well to a change in the diet and the principles of the Liver Cleansing Diet found on *pages 20 to 27* need to be followed for life. I have had several patients with this problem who have been able to return their liver function to normal, after adopting my diet. However, they have found that the liver function becomes abnormal again if they do not maintain the liver diet principles. Avoid all dairy products (milk, butter, cheese, cream, yoghurt, icecream), preserved meats, fried foods and fatty meats. Pay careful attention to any drugs or medications because they may aggravate your liver inflammation. Check with your doctor before taking them.

It is also important to take natural anti-inflammatory supplements to reduce the inflammation in the bile ducts. The most important ones are the antioxidant vitamins, vitamin C, E and natural beta-carotene. Selenium exerts a powerful anti-inflammatory effect and the dosage required is 200mcg daily. I recommend that you take a designer yeast powder high in selenium and its synergistic trace minerals, in a dose of 2 teaspoons daily. Raw vegetable juices, containing a mixture of carrot, celery, beetroot, broccoli and apple provide many benefits. Foods high in sulphur such as garlic, onions, legumes and eggs enhance sulfation of toxins making them easier to excrete. Cruciferous vegetables such as broccoli, cabbage, cauliflower, kale, mustard greens, radish, bok choy and Brussels sprouts will help liver function and support detoxification pathways.

Primary Biliary Cirrhosis

Primary biliary cirrhosis (PBC) is a disease that attacks the bile ducts in the liver, resulting in their destruction. This causes blockage of the bile ducts so that bile cannot flow freely. Bile builds up in the liver, causing chronic inflammation which leads to scarring of the liver. Scar tissue is the same as collagen, which is thick and fibrous and chokes the liver cells to death. Severe scarring of the liver is called cirrhosis.

PBC affects women around 10 times more frequently than men, probably because of genetic and hormonal factors. It usually develops slowly with symptoms first manifesting in people aged 30 to 60. It is a chronic inflammatory disease and may be autoimmune in origin. PBC may occur in association with other autoimmune diseases such as ulcerative colitis.

This disease has many similarities to sclerosing cholangitis and essentially the dietary and supplement program is the same for both diseases *see page 87*.

As with sclerosing cholangitis, excellent results and long term control of this disease can usually be achieved with nutritional medicine. High doses of vitamin E (1000i.u. twice daily) should be taken to reduce liver scarring. A powerful liver tonic containing natural synergistic nutrients to support liver function should be taken long term. This is available in capsule or powder form.

Liver Transplantation

This is the procedure whereby the healthy liver of a donor is used to replace the diseased liver of a recipient. It is often very successful and between 70 and 80% of recipients of a transplanted liver are alive 12 months after the operation. Most of these 12-month survivors become long term survivors. Lifelong immunosuppressant drugs must be taken after a liver transplant. All patients under the age of 65 with advanced cirrhosis are candidates for a liver transplant.

How can I Boost My Metabolism and Banish Cellulite?

Cellulite is a stubborn problem for many people and is far more common in women. Even women who are not overweight may suffer with cellulite. If you have cellulite do not become depressed as it can gradually be eliminated by easy and proven techniques to improve your metabolism. Cellulite is the term used to describe the build up of irregular, lumpy fat deposits typically around the buttocks, hips and thighs. Cellulite has an "orange peel" appearance because the overlying skin is dimpled. The key to eradicating cellulite and keeping it off is found in restoring a healthy metabolism!

What is metabolism?

Metabolism is the term used to describe the inner chemical processes of the cells during which food energy is turned into cellular energy.

The rate at which this happens is called the metabolic rate. If you have a high metabolic rate your cells will convert food energy into cellular energy quickly, which means that you will not gain weight easily. Conversely if you have a low metabolic rate, you will not convert food energy into cellular energy efficiently and food energy will be stored in the form of body fat. It is well recognized that metabolism has a lot to do with excessive weight gain and those with a slow or sluggish metabolism will gain weight very easily and tend to develop cellulite. Fat cells in areas of cellulite have a very low metabolic rate and this is why it is so hard to burn fat off from these affected areas.

What Controls the Metabolic Rate?

A. The Liver

A healthy liver is the major fat burning organ in the body and regulates fat metabolism in several very sophisticated ways. In simple terms we can describe the liver as an organ which can burn unwanted body fat, or pump excessive fat out of the body through the bile into the intestines.

Many people who develop cellulite have an underlying problem with their liver function. In such cases the liver has turned from a fat burner into a fat storer, and we see fatty deposits building up in the liver itself. It is as if the liver has become a warehouse for fat.

Improving the liver function is essential to eradicate cellulite.

B. The Thyroid Gland

The thyroid gland produces the hormone called thyroxine, also known as T4. Thyroxine is not an active hormone and must be converted inside the body cells to its active form called Triiodothyronine or T3.

T3 acts directly upon the energy factories inside the cells (mitochondria), to speed up the rate at which they convert food energy into physical energy. In other words T3 speeds up the metabolic rate.

The thyroid gland can be considered to be the throttle or accelerator of body metabolism.

The conversion of T4 into T3 can slow down with advancing years, poor diet, or exposure to various toxins such as excessive alcohol or insecticides. This is called "thyroid resistance" and results in abnormally low levels of T3. People with low levels of T3 will have a very slow metabolic rate and will age more rapidly. They will experience fluid retention, dryness of the skin and hair, easy weight gain and a tendency to puffy cellulite. It is easy to check the levels of the T4 and T3 hormones with a simple blood test that your local doctor can arrange.

Factors that increase Cellulite

• Sluggish metabolic rate caused by imbalances in the function of the thyroid gland and liver.

• Build up of toxins in the fat cells. These toxins overload the energy factories inside the fat cells, which reduces their ability to burn fat. Most of these toxins are fat-soluble and only the liver can turn fat soluble toxins into water-soluble toxins. If this does not occur the toxins cannot be eliminated from the body and will stay inside the fat cells. This will lead to persistence of cellulite.

• Hormonal changes which occur during pregnancy and the premenstrual phase of the cycle. Many women complain of weight gain and increased cellulite before menstrual bleeding, and during and after pregnancy. This can be prevented by correct diet and keeping your metabolism at efficient levels.

• Lack of exercise, which will reduce blood supply to the fatty areas and increase fluid retention in cellulite areas. We recommend swimming, cycling and brisk walking.

• Eating the wrong types of fats, which increases the workload of the liver. These "heavy fats" tend to accumulate inside the fat cells causing the cells to become hard and swollen. It is as if these fat cells become choked with fat, which slows down the metabolic processes inside the fat cells. These hard swollen fat cells then become trapped by connective tissues, which makes them irregular and lumpy in appearance. This gives the appearance of cellulite. It is vital to avoid these "heavy fats" if you want to eradicate cellulite.

The fats to avoid are found in:
Deep Fried foods
Processed foods and snack foods containing hydrogenated vegetable oils
Fatty parts of animal meats
Chicken skin and pork crackling
 Preserved meats such as ham, bacon, sausage, pizza meats,etc
Smoked meats and delicatessen meats
Margarine and oils that are not cold pressed
Dairy products (milk, butter, cheese, cream, chocolate, icecream and yoghurt)
Foods containing dairy products as additives

To avoid these types of fats may necessitate quite a few changes in your diet, however you will find that this is easy to stick to. The principles of the Liver Cleansing Diet found on *pages 20 to 27* of this book, give you the correct guidelines to follow. The good news is that you will not be hungry while avoiding these fatty foods because you will be able to eat and enjoy the good fats which are the "light fats". The good fats will give you a feeling of fullness and satisfaction while boosting energy and enhancing metabolism. The good fats are known as essential fatty acids and have not been processed in any way. They must be fresh to be beneficial for health.

Examples of foods containing the good fats are:
Cold pressed seed and vegetable oils
Raw nuts and seeds
Legumes (beans, peas, lentils)
Seafood (fresh or canned)
Spirulina, evening primrose oil, borage oil, lecithin
Many fruits and vegetables, especially egg plant, bananas and green-leafy vegetables.
Nut and seed spreads (eg. tahini, almond paste, and humous)
Eggs in moderation (say around 6 per week) are safe. These are allowed because although they contain some cholesterol, it is combined with lecithin and sulfur bearing amino acids,which help the liver to burn fat.
If you want to eradicate cellulite obtain your fats from our list of good fats, and avoid the "hard fats" in the first list. You will be surprised just how easy and effective this is. The essential fatty acids found in the "good fat foods" will keep your fat cells soft and flexible and give them healthy

cell membranes. This will enhance energy flow inside and across the cell membranes, which will keep the metabolic rate inside the fat cells at a high level. This will prevent the fat cells from becoming swollen and hard with excessive fats. Your fat cells will remain soft, flexible and of normal size, and therefore cellulite cannot develop.

Your Body Type and Cellulite
There are 4 different body types:
Android, Gynaeoid, Thyroid and Lymphatic *(see below)*

These 4 body types have unique hormonal and metabolic characteristics. Some body types gain weight easily and are also more susceptible to cellulite. In all body types the above guidelines concerning the good (light) fats and the bad (heavy) fats can be followed to eradicate cellulite. The supplements discussed to enhance fat burning and metabolism will be effective for cellulite in all the body types because they work on the cellular level.

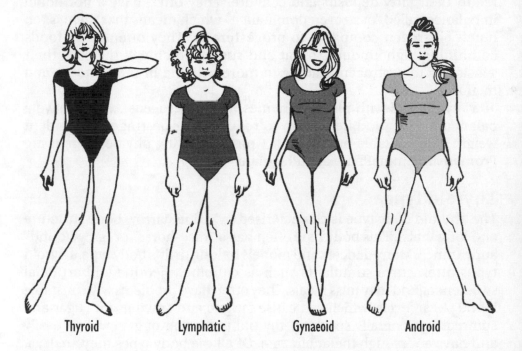

Thyroid   Lymphatic   Gynaeoid   Android

Android Type
The Android body type has broad shoulders and strong muscular limbs. The trunk is somewhat straight up and down and there is not much of a waist. The pelvis is narrow and the hips do not flare. Android types have an anabolic metabolism, which means that they tend to be "body-

building" and will gain weight in the upper part of their body so that they may become apple-shaped. Most of their weight gain occurs on the front of the abdomen. They build muscle mass easily and make good athletes. They tend to produce more male hormones than do the other body types. Android types tend to crave foods that are high in cholesterol and salt. The body turns cholesterol into steroid hormones, which will have a body building effect. This may lead to some cellulite in the abdominal area, trunk and upper buttocks, but not below the hips.

Gynaeoid Type

The Gynaeoid body type is the curvy shape with small to medium shoulders tapering to a small waist and then flaring below to wide curvaceous hips. Weight gain occurs only on the thighs and lower buttocks and gives a very feminine and curvy shape. Many gynaeoid types will have a big problem with cellulite accumulating around the upper thighs and buttocks. If they try to lose weight with just any old low-fat low-calorie diet, it can be quite frustrating because weight will tend to come off easily from areas where there is not a problem, while the thighs and buttocks retain their fatty deposits and cellulite. They often have a hormonal imbalance called "oestrogen dominance" which means that there is too much oestrogen compared to progesterone. They often crave foods combining high amounts of fat and sugar, which will increase their sensitivity to oestrogen, leading to more cellulite in the buttocks and thighs.

They do well with plant hormones (phytoestrogens), which have a balancing effect and help them to reduce their oestrogen dependent weight gain. Suitable products for women wanting phytoestrogens are Promensil, FemmePhase and PhytoLife.

Thyroid Type

The Thyroid body type is characterised by a fine narrow bone structure and long limbs. This body type often has a "race-horse" or "grey hound" appearance. Many dancers and models belong to this body type. Thyroid types often crave stimulants such as caffeine, nicotine and artificial sweeteners, and may miss meals. They often have problems with unstable blood sugar levels, which can cause fatigue and cravings for sugar and stimulants. Generally speaking, thyroid types do not gain weight easily and have a very high metabolic rate. Of all the body types they are least likely to develop cellulite and if it does occur, it is on the buttocks and back of the thighs.

Lymphatic Types

Lymphatic body types gain weight all over the body, and have a "cuddly baby doll" appearance. Weight gain occurs very easily because lymphatic types have a very low metabolic rate. They also have a dysfunctional lymphatic system resulting in generalised fluid retention, which makes them look fatter than they are. They are prone to deposits of fat swollen with lymphatic fluid, which can cause severe cellulite. This type of cellulite gives them thick puffy limbs so that it is hard to see their bone structure. They often avoid exercise and crave dairy products, both of which will exacerbate their cellulite.

In The Past

Years ago it was recognised that there were different body types and they were categorised according to their shape only. This was before we understood the hormonal and metabolic differences between the body types. For your interest, just in case you find them in some old textbook I will describe them for you.

Android   was called the mesomorph
Thyroid   was called the ectomorph
Lymphatic was called the endomorph
Gynaeoid   this body type was not described, probably being considered a combination of several types.

Natural Supplements to Help Metabolism

These will stimulate fat burning and reduce cellulite.

A. Improve Liver Function

This will increase the ability of the liver to burn fat and pump fat out of the body through the bile. It will also help to breakdown fat-soluble toxins that would otherwise become trapped in the fatty tissues and lead to cellulite. Liver tonics are the most effective strategy, however you will need a powerful tonic that can really improve liver function. I recommend a liver tonic powder or capsules that contain B vitamins , anti-oxidants, green tea, zinc, lecithin, cruciferous vegetable powder, and the amino acids taurine, cysteine, glutamine, and glycine, plus the powerful liver herb called St. Mary's Thistle. Dosage is one teaspoon mixed in juice twice daily or two capsules twice daily. Eat raw fruits and vegetables with every meal and drink at least 8 glasses (2litres/4 pints) of filtered water everyday.

B. Improve Thyroid Function

The thyroid gland has a high requirement for trace minerals because the enzymes that produce thyroid hormone (T4) and convert it to the active form (T3) are dependent upon trace minerals. The most important minerals for this process are selenium, zinc, manganese and iodine. Many people with cellulite have a deficiency of trace minerals, which leads to sluggish thyroid function and a low metabolic rate. To boost trace minerals I recommend that you include in the diet unprocessed grains, nuts, seeds and legumes.

I have found that an excellent way to boost trace minerals needed by the thyroid gland, is to take designer yeast powders enhanced with these minerals. They are a food supplement that contains an easily absorbed form of organic minerals. A good designer yeast powder should contain selenium, chromium, molybdenum, zinc, manganese, magnesium, calcium, vegetable powders (also high in trace minerals), and the herb kelp (very high in trace minerals). Some yeast powders also contain the natural ingredient (usually extracted from apples) called Malic acid, which helps the cells to turn food energy into physical energy. Generally speaking you will require two teaspoons of these powders daily to obtain these benefits. Stir the powder into water or juice and take with meals. Selemite B tablets can be taken as an alternative to powders.

C. Stimulate your Fat Cells to Burn Fat

These natural substances will help you to burn fat safely without drug induced side effects. An effective natural weight loss tablet called METABOCEL contains the following ingedients:

- Tyrosine - 100mg three times daily before meals.
- Brindleberry - (Garcinia quaesita) 5500mg (extra strength) which is the richest source of Hydroxy Citric Acid (HCA), three times daily before meals.
- Kelp - 25mg three times daily before meals.
- Vitamin B6 - 10mg three times daily before meals.
- Zinc amino acid chelate, chromium picolinate and capsicum extract are able to enhance the effect of tyrosine and brindleberry.

Actions: Natural substances, which eliminate cellulite and reduce weight scientifically, must be able to do the following:
Stimulate thyroid function
Stimulate brown fat metabolism
Reduce sugar cravings
Stabilise blood sugar levels
Boost energy

Tyrosine is a precursor of the energy hormones thyroxine and adrenalin. Tyrosine stimulates thyroid gland function and therefore metabolism. Tyrosine is needed by the thyroid gland to manufacture thyroid hormones. It reduces brain fatigue and improves mood.
Kelp is a sea herb and is an excellent source of trace minerals, especially iodine, which is required to make thyroid hormone. Kelp contains many trace minerals needed by the body and is an excellent aid to general health.

Kelp contains organic iodine and is not a problem for those allergic to inorganic iodine. It is beneficial for the glandular system, especially the thyroid, pituitary and adrenal glands.

Brindleberry is a fruit used for centuries by the people of Asia because it enhances the flavour and satisfaction of meals. The rind of this fruit is rich in Hydroxy Citric Acid (HCA). The most effective dose of brindleberry is 5,500mg, 3 times daily, taken just before food. Brindleberry is more effective if it is combined with tyrosine, kelp, vitamin B6, zinc, chromium and capsicum and this is why METABOCEL is a synergistic formula.

HCA is proven to naturally suppress the appetite and stop the production of new fat. HCA from Brindleberry is clinically proven to help inhibit the production of fat by blocking the enzyme that causes fat to be stored by the body. So while your losing weight you are also halting the formation of new fat. **Ref 18.**

All these natural ingredients are available combined together in METABOCEL. For more information on natural fat burning nutrients see your local pharmacy or health food store, or call the Health Advisory Service on (612) 4653 1445 or Fax: (612) 4653 1144 or visit www.whas.com.au

Avoid artificial stimulants, artificial sweeteners, amphetamine type drugs and the herb Ephedra, because these things will temporarily hype up your metabolic rate and reduce your appetite. However once you stop them your system has become dependent upon them and you will probably feel tired, depressed and very hungry. The worst thing of all is that when you come off these stimulants your metabolic rate will be temporarily lower than ever and you will gain weight rapidly.

The natural fat burners that I have discussed have a balancing effect upon the overall metabolism. They will not cause any dramatic changes in your metabolic rate, which is good, otherwise you will become a yoyo dieter and will get bigger over the long term.

If you have queries concerning your weight, body type, metabolism or cellulite why not phone us at the

Health Advisory Service on (612) 4653 1445 or (612) 9387 8111.
We have a naturopath Robyn Spillane available for consultation. Robyn Spillane works closely with Dr. Sandra Cabot and does regular free consultations in health food stores and pharmacies in Sydney.
You may also visit our web site @ http://www.whas.com.au
We have an interactive web site that will enable you to work out your body type by doing our body type questionnaire. Further information is available in Dr. Sandra Cabot's book called "The Body Shaping Diet."

Appendix - Section One

Tests For Liver Function

Most of the standard or routine blood tests that your doctor will order to check "liver function" are in reality only able to detect liver disease. These tests are not sensitive enough to accurately reflect liver function. These tests will usually be abnormal in liver disease, however they can still give normal readings in some cases of significant liver disease. This is why it is important for you to consult a specialist in liver diseases (hepatologist), if you suspect that your liver is unhealthy and yet conventional blood tests remain normal.

A routine blood test for liver function will be processed by an automated multichannel analyser, and will check the blood levels of the following :-

<u>Total Bilirubin</u> - Normal range is 3 - 18 umol/L (0.174 - 1.04mg/dL).

Liver Enzymes

AST - (aspartate aminotransferase) which was previously called SGOT. This enzyme can also be elevated in heart and muscular diseases and is not liver specific. Normal range of AST is 5-45 U/L.

ALT - (alanine aminotransferase) which was previously called SGPT and is more specific for liver damage. Normal range of ALT is 5-45 U/L.

AP - (alkaline phosphatase) is elevated in many types of liver disease but also in non-liver related diseases. Normal range of AP is 30-120 U/L.

GT - (gamma glutamyl transpeptidase) is often elevated in those who use alcohol or other liver toxic substances to excess. Normal range of GT is 5-35 U/L.

The reason why all or some of these enzymes become elevated in cases of liver disease is that they are normally contained inside the liver cells (hepatocytes). They only leak into the blood stream when the liver cells are damaged. Thus measuring liver enzymes is only able to detect liver damage and does not measure liver function in a sensitive way.

Blood Proteins (manufactured by the liver)

Total protein- Normal range is 60-80 g/L (6 - 8g/dL).

> **Serum albumin** - Normal range is 30-50 g/L (3 -5 g/dL). Serum albumin is a good guide to the severity of chronic liver disease. A healthy liver manufactures the protein albumin, and falling levels show deteriorating liver function.
>
> **Gamma globulin** protein levels may be abnormal in chronic liver disease.
>
> **Prothrombin time** assesses the ability of the liver to manufacture clotting factors.

Functional Tests of the Liver

Recently tests that assess the liver's function, especially its detoxification abilities, have become available. These tests are called Functional Liver Challenge Tests or a Functional Liver Detoxification Profile. During these tests the liver is challenged with caffeine, aspirin and paracetamol in safe oral doses. Samples of urine and saliva are then collected at timed intervals and sent to the laboratory where their levels of the excreted forms of these drugs are measured. These tests are non-invasive and assess the ability of the liver to detoxify and eliminate drugs and other chemicals. These tests are unique in that they assess the functional capacity of the liver in both phase one and phase two detoxification pathways. They can be conducted in the patient's home and are simple to perform. Your health care practitioner can arrange them for you.

These specialised tests are available from:

> **Analytical Reference Laboratories Pty Ltd (ARL),**
> **5 Leveson Street, North Melbourne, Victoria 3051 Australia**
> **Phone: (613) 9328 3586   Fax: (613) 9326 5004**
>
> **The Great Smokies Laboratories**
> **18A Regent Park Boulevarde, Ashville**
> **North Carolina, USA, 28806**
> **Phone: (828) 285 2223**

Liver Help Resources

AUSTRALIA
Hepatitis C Councils of Australia
(They have excellent regular magazines on Hepatitis C)

Victorian Council
Level 9, Carlow House, 289 Flinders Lane, Melbourne Vic. 3000
Phone: (613) 9639 3200 or 1800 703 003

NSW Council
P.O. Box 432, Darlinghurst NSW 1300.
Phone: (612) 9332 1599 or 1800 803 990

Health Advisory Service
P.O. Box 54, Cobbitty NSW 2570
Phone: (612) 4653 1445   Fax: (612) 4653 1144
Email: cabot@ozemail.com.au

Australian Gastroenterology Institute
145 Macquarie St, Sydney, NSW, 2000
Phone–: (612) 9256 5455 Fax: (612) 9241 4586

Children's Liver Alliance
23 Dirkale St, Mansfield, QLD, 4122

UK
British Liver Trust
Central House, Central Avenue, Ransomes Europark
Ipswich IP3 9QG
Phone: (44) 1473 276326 and (44) 1473 276328
E-mail: info@liver-t.demon.co.uk

Children's Liver Disease Foundation
138 Digbeth, Birmingham B5 6DR
Phone: (44) 121 643 7282

USA
American Association for the Study of Liver Diseases (AASLD)
6900 Grove Rd, Thorofare, NJ, USA, 08086
Phone: (609) 848-1000

American Liver Foundation (ALF)
1425 Pompton Ave, Cedar Grove, NJ, USA, 07009

Phone: 1-800- Go Liver (1-800 465-4837)

Hepatitis Foundation International (HFI)
30 Sunrise Terrace, Cedar Grove, NJ, USA, 07009-1423
Phone: 1-800-891-0707

Hepatitis B Foundation
700 E. Butler Ave, Doylestown, PA, USA, 18901
Phone: (215) 489-4900

Hepatitis C Foundation
1502 Russett Drive, Warminster, PA, USA, 18974
Phone: (215) 672-2606 Fax: (215) 672-1518

National Digestive Diseases Information
Clearing House, 2 Information Way
Bethesda, MD, USA, 20892-3570
Phone: (301) 654-3810

Helpful Web Sites

Health Advisory Service
http://www.liverdoctor.com

American Liver Foundation
http://sadieo.ucsf.edu/ALF/alffinal/homepagealf.html
and http://www.liverfoundation.org

HepNet
http://www.hepnet.com/

AASLD
http://hepar-sfgh.ucsf.edu/

HFI
http://www.hepfi.org

Hepatitis B Foundation
http://www2.hepb.org/hepb/

Hepatitis C Foundation
http://www.hepcfoundation.org

Section Two - The Bowel

Chapter One - How to have a Healthy Bowel
    Causes of Bowel Dysfunction ...104
    Strategies to Help Bowel Disorders ...105
    Natural Remedies for the Bowel ...110
    Bowel Parasites - A Case History ...111

Chapter Two - Bowel Problems
    Constipation ...114
    Laxatives ...114
    Megacolon ...115
    Inflammatory Bowel Disease ...117
        Ulcerative Colitis ...117
        Crohn's Disease ...119
    Irritable Bowel Syndrome ...121
    Dietary Fibre ...124
    Prolapsed Colon ...126
    Peptic Ulcer ...127
    Reflux ...130
    Coeliac Disease ...131
        Gluten Free Diet ...132
    Haemorrhoids ...135
    Diverticulitis ...136
    Bowel Cancer ...138
    Bowel Polyps ...139
    Recovery from Bowel Cancer - a patient's story ...141

Chapter Three - Digestive and Related Problems ...145
    Candida ...147
    High Cholesterol ...150
    Pancreatitis ...151
    Diabetes ...155
    Food Allergies

Appendix Section Two:
    Tests for Bowel and Digestive Function ...158
    Colonoscopy ...159
    Sigmoidoscopy ...159
    Barium Enema ...159
    High Salicylate Foods ...160

Chapter One - How to Have a Healthy Bowel

What is the Digestive System?

Simply put, the digestive tract consists of a long tube, which connects the mouth to the anus. After food is swallowed it passes through the oesophagus to the stomach, where it is churned up with acid and stomach enzymes into small particles. This then passes into the small intestine, which is around 20 feet long. The most important function of the small intestine is to digest and absorb nutrients from the food particles that arrive from the stomach. In the upper part of the small intestine, secretions from the liver and gallbladder (bile), and the pancreas (enzymes), are inserted through a small tube (duct), situated near the pancreas gland. *See colour diagram between pages 32 and 33.* The term bowel is synonymous with intestine.

The small intestines are referred to as the small bowel. The small bowel has 3 parts. The part nearest the stomach is called the duodenum, the next part is the jejunum and the third part is the ileum, which connects with the large intestine. Where the ileum joins the large bowel (at the caecal area of the colon), there is a valve called the ileocaecal valve. *See diagram on page 104.* This valve is designed to stop food particles and faeces from refluxing backwards into the ileum. The ileum is a vitally important part of the small intestine because it is here that the essential vitamin B 12 and bile salts are absorbed. If the ileum becomes diseased as in Crohn's disease, severe nutritional deficiencies can result leading to serious diseases.

The large intestines or large bowel are divided into the colon and the rectum. The first part of the colon has a sac like shape and is called the caecum, which is the site of attachment of the appendix. The colon has an upside down U shape, and goes from the ascending colon to the transverse colon to the descending colon, and finally the sigmoid colon, which joins the rectum. The main function of the colon is the absorption of water from the processed food residue that arrives after essential nutrients have been absorbed in the small intestine. The last part of the large bowel is the rectum, which is a reservoir for faeces, which are stored until the urge to pass a bowel motion is felt. Problems can occur if the size of the colon becomes too large, or if it develops inflammation, spasm or pockets (diverticula) in its muscular walls. These are common problems in people who consume the typical Western diet.

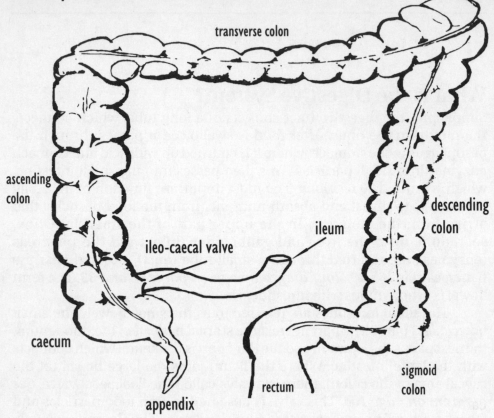

transverse colon

ascending
colon

descending
colon

ileum

ileo-caecal valve

caecum

sigmoid
colon

rectum

appendix

Causes of Bowel Dysfunction

There are many problems that can affect the small and large intestines, and most are associated with incorrect dietary habits and/or an overgrowth or infestation with unfriendly microorganisms in the bowels.

Stress also plays a large role in the function of the bowels because it can reduce the circulation of blood to the absorptive areas of the bowels.

The adequacy of liver and pancreatic function is also important because dysfunction of either organ can lead to poor digestion of food and reduced assimilation of nutrients. Thus even though you may be eating a reasonably good diet, you can suffer with malnutrition because the essential nutrients are not being absorbed from the gut.

The problems of Irritable Bowel Syndrome, Spastic Colon, Constipation, Ulcerative Colitis, Crohn's disease, and offensive gas and wind, often all share these common factors to a varying degree. It is only the severity of the inflammation and the area of the bowel that it attacks, which determines what type of bowel disorder will manifest.

Strategies to help all types of Bowel Disorders:

1. Maintain a Healthy Population of Microorganisms in your Bowel.

It is important to be aware that your bowels may be harbouring excessive populations of unfriendly microorganisms such as fungi (most commonly yeasts such as candida albicans), bacteria, viruses and parasites. The term parasite is used to describe a great variety of creatures that vary in complexity from single celled organisms, all the way up to worms that may be several inches or longer. Common disease causing parasites are Giardia lambia, Entamoeba histolytica, Blastocystis hominis and Cryptosporidium, which can be very difficult to detect with routine stool analysis and cultures. When a stool specimen is examined for parasites many of the yeasts that are seen are already dead. Stool cultures therefore often fail to reveal the presence of fungi even when the gut is heavily infected. Some laboratories *(see page 99)* will examine repeated fresh stool specimens obtained after inducing mild diarrhoea with laxatives and this will increase the chances of detection.

Those who suffer with an overgrowth of unhealthy microorganisms in the bowels are said to have "intestinal dysbiosis".

It can be difficult to eradicate intestinal parasites completely and many sufferers find that they keep on recurring. I have found that a medication called Niciosamide (brand name Yomesan) is the most effective remedy against tape worm and roundworms. Unfortunately this remedy is no longer marketed in Australia, however for those who have chronic problems with intestinal worms, you can contact the manufacturing company which is Bayer Australia. They may be able to help you.

A natural anti-parasite remedy that can sometimes be quite helpful is called "Rainbow Herbal Worming" and is a liquid combination of herbs such as artemisia vulgaris and aloe bardens leaf. It is taken four times a day for 3 days.

Anti-parasitic remedies are often more effective if they are followed by a purge, during which many dead parasites will be expelled in the faeces. To achieve the required laxative effect you can take 1 to 2 teaspoons of epsom salts with four glasses of water, two hours after finishing the anti-parasitic medication.

To reduce bowel infections with unfriendly bacteria, parasites and yeasts:

- **Avoid** refined sugars and carbohydrates as this is fuel for microorganisms especially yeasts
- **Avoid** preserved foods, especially meats (pizza meats, corned beef,

ham, devon, bacon, sausage, smoked meats and smoked fish etc)
• **Avoid** mouldy or pickled foods such as old peanuts, green potatoes, dried fruits that are moudly or bitter and yeast extracts.
• **Avoid** long term use of antibiotic and steroid drugs.
• **Eat** plentiful fibre in the form of raw vegetables and fruits, wholegrain, bran, ground seeds and legumes, raw or lightly cooked sweetcorn. This will have a "broom effect" and sweep the walls of the colon removing layers of encrusted and hardened faeces, which harbour unfriendly microorganisms.
• **Use** a fibre powder regularly to cleanse the colon - *see suitable formula page 115*
• **Follow** practises of good hygiene *(see page 25)*
• **Use** natural antibiotics to kill intestinal yeasts, bacteria and parasites. Natural antibiotic foods, herbs and condiments are cabbage juice, cruciferous vegetables (cabbage, cauliflower, Brussels sprouts, broccoli), raw garlic, onions, leeks, radishes, fenugreek, gingerroot, hot chilli, lemon juice, tumeric, mustard and rosemary.

The most powerful natural antibiotic for the gut is, you guessed it, RAW garlic. Oh no you say, not that again! If you can manage to eat 4 to 6 cloves everyday for 4 weeks you will be amazed at the creatures that can be eradicated and expelled from your bowels. Garlic is able to kill bacteria, parasites and yeasts. If you have a large overgrowth, even higher doses may be required. Raw garlic cloves can be grated, chopped very finely or pressed in a garlic press, and then mixed well throughout your cooked food and salads. It tastes nicer with some cold pressed olive oil and apple cider vinegar. Raw onions and leeks also have valuable antibiotic effects in the bowel, and if you cannot tolerate garlic you may find that these things work well for you.

Take supplements of Lactobacillus acidophilus (must be refrigerated), or use unflavoured soy yoghurts high in this friendly bacteria. This friendly bacterium fights the bad bacteria and helps to maintain ecological balance. It is particularly good after antibiotic therapy.

Some naturopaths recommend tea or powder from Pau d'arco bark to fight yeast infections, while others recommend the 8-carbon fatty acid called Caprylic acid which is safe and may help in mild cases.

Typical herbs used to destroy and expel worms from the body are black walnut hulls, chaparral, cloves, liquorice, gentian and wormwood.

The herb Olive Leaf extract is very helpful in fighting an overgrowth of yeast and parasites, as well as bacteria and viruses in the bowel, and doses range from 500 to 1000mg (of a 10% extract), three times daily just before meals.

Those who are frequent international travellers are more at risk from infections such as hepatitis B and gut infections, and although vaccinations against many of these things are available today, it is still wise to protect your liver and immune system so that they can cope with this increased challenge. Practise good hygiene, avoid contaminated water supplies, and boil your water. While travelling take a good liver tonic, garlic and olive leaf extract capsules to fight these unfriendly bugs while they are still in your gut, and before they get a chance to damage your liver.

2. Improve Dietary Habits

One of the most important and yet often overlooked strategies to improve bowel function for all people, is to drink more pure WATER. I cannot tell you how many people I have seen over the years with bowel problems who are chronically dehydrated. This causes the bowel contents to harden and stagnate, which can lead to overgrowth of bacteria and inflammation of the bowel lining. I recommend at least 2 litres of pure water daily, and in those with inflammatory bowel diseases up to 3 litres may be required everyday.

By following the principles of the Liver Cleansing Diet, *see pages 20 to 27*, you will have the basic tools for a diet that is conducive to healthy bowels.

Many people lack fibre because they eat refined sugars and carbohydrates, and too much animal meat and dairy products. Without fibre, the contents of the bowel will stagnate, which can lead to inflammation from excessive toxin formation. Lack of fibre will also force the bowel muscles to contract too strongly in an effort to move the faeces along to the rectum to stimulate a bowel movement. These excessive contractions will increase the pressure inside the bowel, which leads to spastic colon and the formation of pockets in the bowel wall (diverticula). *See diagram on page 137*.

Avoid excess alcohol as this can cause inflammation of the bowel wall. In some people alcohol causes a form of colitis and must be avoided completely. Avoid gastric irritants such as excess coffee and cigarettes.

Thirty to forty percent of the diet should consist of RAW vegetables and fruits, with the ratio of vegetables to fruits being 4 to 1. In severe cases of candida it may be necessary to greatly reduce the amount of fruits and increase raw vegetables.

Raw foods contain living enzymes, antibiotics and phytonutrients that improve digestion, fight unfriendly microorganisms and reduce inflammation of the bowel wall. We have plenty of yummy salad recipes to keep you entertained.

For some it can be very hard to change old dietary habits and a new perspective may be needed. This was the case for Eric, a 52 year old bachelor who came to see me complaining of excessive weight gain, abdominal bloating, fatigue, sore joints and indigestion. He had been fully investigated and the only problem found was a fatty liver. He was a typical bachelor and that, combined with his high powered career of accounting, left him no spare time to follow a complicated dietary regime. He felt so unwell that he knew he had to change but the task was overwhelming to him. He lived on take away convenience and fast foods high in fat and sugar and did not go shopping.

I counselled him about the foods in the Liver Cleansing Diet, telling him that he should try to follow its vital principles, and to pick and choose the recipes that were easy for him to prepare and enjoy. With a mammoth effort Eric started to visit green grocers, butchers and super markets to source the foods that his liver needed to repair itself. After 8 weeks he returned and was happy to report that he felt much better and was losing weight easily. He had increased his energy levels and his mind was much sharper and clearer. He did however complain that the busy time of the year was approaching and that he could not see himself finding the time to continue shopping and preparing food. I suggested that he hire a woman that could come to his home 2 or 3 days a week and shop, and prepare his meals that could be refrigerated and stored hygienically. At first he complained that this would be expensive, however after we worked out the cost of continually eating out he could see that he would actually save money and precious time. He would be able to pack a lunch to take to work from the food that the cook had left for him. This way he would have control over what he ate and be able to enjoy home cooked meals. I am happy to say that this worked out very well for him and he is continuing to improve and lose weight.

3. Improve Digestion and Absorption of Nutrients from Food.

Chew food thoroughly and have teeth and jaw problems checked out early. Do not eat very much if you are angry or stressed and do not over eat.

Drink only small amounts with meals because fluids will dilute the gastric juices needed for digestion. The lining of the stomach produces hydrochloric acid, which provides the correct acidity for the digestive enzymes, pepsin and rennin, as well as those secreted in the small intestines to break down food. Hydrochloric acid is also required for efficient liberation of the important nutrient vitamin B 12.

Deficiency of stomach hydrochloric acid is common in those over 60 years of age, and can lead to weakened digestion and deficiency of vitamin B 12. In these cases it is desirable to increase stomach hydrochloric acid, and this can be done with tablets of Betaine Hydrochloride. The usual dose is between 60 to 500 mg of Betaine Hydrochloride taken in the middle of a meal. Once dissolved in the stomach Betaine Hydrochloride yields 25% of its weight as hydrochloric acid. Another tablet to increase hydrochloric acid is

Glutamic acid Hydrochloride, which is slightly less potent and requires a dose of 600 to 1800 mg during meals. Those with a severe deficiency of stomach hydrochloric acid, known as Achlorhydria, may have an increased risk of stomach cancer and for this reason antioxidants such as vitamin C, E and selenium should be part of the daily supplementation program.

Another useful technique to increase stomach acidity during a meal is to sip a glass of water containing 2 to 3 tablespoons of good quality organic apple cider vinegar with the juice of half a lemon added. Some people find that this practise really improves their digestion and reduces flatulence and abdominal bloating.

If you find that you feel uncomfortable after eating a regular or large sized meal it is most worthwhile to try a supplement containing digestive enzymes. The pancreas produces vital enzymes called proteases, lipase and amylase, without which it is impossible to breakdown proteins, fats and carbohydrates. It is not uncommon for a slight to moderate deficiency of these pancreatic enzymes to occur, especially in those over 50 years of age. Lack of these enzymes will result in poor breakdown of proteins, fats and carbohydrates, leaving only partially digested food to pass through the bowel. This reduces absorption of vital nutrients from the lining of the gut and malnutrition of some degree will result. Furthermore only partially digested proteins will be absorbed from the gut, which will overload the liver and may cause allergies. The growth of unfriendly microorganisms is more common inside intestines containing only partially digested foods.

The most powerful way to take the full complement of digestive enzymes is in the form of some type of whole pancreas preparation, which comes from animal sources. Such a suitable preparation is called Pancreatin and the dosage is 2 - 4 grams with each meal. If you do not like the thought of taking animal pancreas or you are a vegan, you may want to try a digestive preparation which contains enzymes from the fungus aspergillus niger. This excellent product is available in the USA and is called TYME-ZYME .

Enzymes are available without a prescription in tablet, capsule, powder and liquid forms. For maximum effectiveness the enzyme supplement you choose should contain all of the major enzyme groups - amylase, lipase and protease. You can also make your own digestive enzymes by drying papaya seeds and grinding them in a coffee grinder into a powder. Sprinkle the powder onto your food and it gives a slight peppery taste. Keep your enzyme supplements in a cool dry place to ensure potency. As we grow older the ability of the body to produce enzymes diminishes, and enzyme supplements can make a huge improvement to the digestive and nutritional health of persons over 50 years of age.

The body can also obtain enzymes from ingested food. Unfortunately food enzymes are extremely sensitive to heat, and even low to moderate heat destroys most of the enzymes in foods. This is one of the reasons I encourage people to eat more raw salads and fruits, as their natural enzyme molecules will improve your digestion and reduce the workload of the liver and pancreas. Foods that are high in enzymes are pineapples, papaya, avocados, mangos and bananas. Sprouts are a potent source of digestive enzymes. Enzymes extracted from papaya and pineapples are available in tablet form and are called papain and bromelain respectively. Although they are proteolytic enzymes and can help with the digestion of proteins, they are not as powerful as a whole pancreatic supplement. When introducing dried beans/legumes into your diet, to avoid unpleasant wind always pre-soak and cook them well. Start with small quantities and gradually build up.

Natural Remedies to help the Bowels

These can be used to increase fibre bulk, soothe irritated mucous linings and reduce muscular spasm in the bowels.

- **Aloe Vera** juice can soothe the lining of the stomach and intestines and is useful for those with stomach ulcers, colitis and irritable bowel syndrome. Occasionally people became allergic to it, so do not use it continually.
- **Psyllium husks** (or powder), are often used as a bowel cleansing fibre and help to remove stagnant waste material from bowel pockets. Like Aloe Vera, some people become allergic to it, so that it causes rashes and itching, so watch out for allergy symptoms if you use it long term.
- **A colon fibre powder** that does not contain gluten or psyllium is called "Fibretone," and is best if you have constipation associated with irritable bowel syndrome, wheat and/or gluten intolerance, bloating or colonic spasm. *See page 115 for formula*
- **Antacids** are often used by those with excess gastric acidity and/or reflux. Avoid the long-term use of antacids containing aluminium. Some simple and harmless antacids are sodium and potassium bicarbonate, magnesium carbonate, magnesium hydroxide and calcium carbonate. Alfalfa juice or alfalfa tablets are alkaline and can soothe gastritis and/or reflux. A brand worth mentioning, that is free of aluminium, is Andrew's Tums.
- **Soothing** and anti-spasm herbs such as golden seal, marshmallow, meadowsweet, valerian, chamomile, peppermint, arrowroot, slippery elm powder will reduce colic and mild bowel inflammation, and benefit those with gastritis.
- **Digestive** herbs such as dandelion, fennel, dill, aniseed, parsley, ginger root and catnip can reduce burping and flatulence.
- **Condiments** that aid digestion and reduce flatulence are caraway, cardamom, coriander, cumin, cloves, gingerroot and tumeric. Tumeric is a liver tonic and the usual dose is 1 - 2 tsp of the powder daily used to flavour food or mixed in juices.

Bowel Parasites

By Trixi Whitmore: *Author of Chemical Free Living*

Here is a summary of my experience with parasites and the beneficial effects of Olive Leaf Extract.

In the 1994 I was diagnosed with "blasto-cystis homminis" found in a stool test and listed as "unknown pathogen" by the testing laboratory. My subsequent research discovered it to be a suspected "protozoa". However it is very widespread in the population and produces symptoms of bloating, flatulence and at times very explosive, smelly loose motions. At first these symptoms were spasmodic, but after a time they seemed to be present most of the time. Although I did not feel ill, I felt extra tired and just not "right"! The doctor did not offer or suggest any treatment. (A subsequent visit to a specialist revealed that there was a severe outbreak in a country town and he was looking for a cure.)

About this time my son, (a young man) suddenly developed symptoms which baffled the doctor. He had been away in Tasmania camping. The symptoms were terrifying and life-threatening. They began with acid indigestion, fatigue and constipation which became worse and worse each day. Antacid preparations were useless. He could eat less and less, had severe rumbling and grumbling in the tummy and the food and drink just seemed to stop at the navel level and took ages to digest. He went into a drugged-like sleep from which it was difficult to wake, and his hands and feet became swollen and very white. His face was ashen. After two weeks he had lost 14 kilograms (30 pounds) and finally when water would not pass through him, he was taken to hospital. Unfortunately it was the weekend and apart from an X ray he had no treatment. However the previous day he had seen a specialist who had prescribed Fasigyn, as he thought it could be giardia. The mixture of Fasigyn with the acute acid caused him agony, as it burnt from the throat down, but eventually after 30 hours, it must have trickled into his intestines as the "blockage" cleared.

After taking Slippery Elm to put a lining back onto his stomach he started eating again, but after three days the symptoms recurred. Flagyl was then prescribed for one week and this brought things back to some kind of normality. However, he had become lactose intolerant and constipated, and had to be careful with food which was difficult to digest. This was a young man who had never had food allergies or bowel irregularities in his whole life.

Over the next 15 months the "bug" keep recurring about every six weeks. Flagyl was useless. I kept finding worm/parasite medicines for him, both herbal and allopathic, some of which worked for a short time, but the "bug" very quickly became immune to the remedy. Over this period I read everything I could about parasites, which I feel are far more prevalent in our country than are recognised! My son consulted various doctors and specialists who did not seem to realise the seriousness of the situation. "Irritable bowel syndrome" was the label! Unfortunately various tests were negative, but no-one stipulated that the most effective stool sample is a PURGED sample.

You might wonder why I have recounted the experience of my son. After 15 months I suddenly developed the same symptoms. (I suspect I may have picked it up while cleaning his toilet and bathroom). My son had another relapse at the same time. After a week of terrible symptoms, when I had lost 6 kilograms (13 pounds), much searching discovered a herbal tapeworm remedy called Rascal, based on chilli. This reversed the situation and our digestion started working again, but alas after three weeks it was ineffective. Further searching found Yomesan (which unfortunately Bayer have recently removed from the Australian market), a tapeworm S2 medicine, which according to their literature is also effective against roundworms.

This worked and saved us from a fate worse than death, and has worked more than once, because it has a different action to other medications. Yomesan treatment is followed by a purge with Epsom salts, which cleans out the dead worms. As you can see we have both been on a roller coaster ride, my son since October 1994 and myself since January 1996.

Because I could not seem to get my digestion or bowels to return to normal, nor to get rid of the parasite problem, I finally found and consulted with a doctor who understood parasite problems. He sent my stool samples to The Great Smokies Laboratories in the USA. (These tests are now available in Australia at Analytical Reference Laboratories Pty Ltd (ARL) 5 Levenson Street, North Melbourne, Victoria 3051 Phone (613) 9328 3586 Fax: (613) 9326 5004

Great Smokies found "blasto-cystis homminis", dientamoeba fragillis (which can be hosted by threadworms), and dysbiosis (unhealthy microorganisms in the gut), rated at 12 on a scale of 1-10. Such was the health of my gut!

A long period of convalescence has now taken place with intermittent doses of Yomesan and other remedies, and I hope that both my son and I are beating the problem. All along I suspected that my son had something "different" - a very virulent "bug" which behaved in a different way to anything in the parasite literature, but responded to parasite medication. (I must thank Bayer for supplying me with such useful information on various parasites.)

After so many negative stool tests, I decided to start looking myself for evidence of worms. The ideal time was after dosing with Yomesan followed by Epsom salts. Persistence paid off, for I found some "interesting items," which I took to a kind and caring naturopath/biochemist who analyses live blood. She has a microscope attached to a colour TV screen. One of the "interesting items" I found was a definite worm, 6mm long, with a heart shaped tail. I photographed it, made a sketch of same, and took it to Newcastle University for identification. *See diagram below.* Also I sent the sketch and particulars to Dr. Leo Galland (world expert on parasites) and The Great Smokies Laboratories. So far no one can identify it! Maybe it is a new species of roundworm? Interestingly two new roundworms have recently been identified, one in Victoria in the muscle tissue of a fireman who was seriously ill, and another named crypto strongulus pulmoni in the sputum of Chronic Fatigue patients in the USA.

I now seem to be on the road to recovery with no evidence of blasto-cystis homminis in recent tests, but do not know just what cured the blasto. Maybe it was the lemon juice and water first thing in the morning. However the dysbiosis was still a problem until a month ago when I tried Olive Leaf Extract. This has had a remarkable effect. The bloating, wind and abnormal motions stopped and for the first time in years everything returned to normal. Heaven! Anyone diagnosed with "irritable bowel syndrome" or parasites should try it.

tail

Worm 6mm long measured by Newcastle University, Department of Parasitology. Classified as "environmental worm"

head

These eggs were visible as I had picked the worm up with tweezers

This was the pattern on the head of the worm

Constipation

The normal frequency of bowel actions varies greatly between people. You should have from one to four bowel actions a day. They should be a brownish colour, be soft and grainy and passed without undue straining. Many of my patients have told me that their stools have changed significantly after commencing the Liver Cleansing Diet. In particular they find that they are softer, easier to pass and much longer. They may contain obvious pieces of undigested vegetables such as sweet corn skins, small parts of plant skins and small parts of leaves. This is a good sign because this increased fibre acts like a broom to cleanse the bowel walls.

Signs to worry about are red blood or a black colour in the stools, or an obvious change in bowel habits from your normal pattern. It is good to look at each bowel action after you pass it to check for general appearance and blood or blackness.

Laxatives

Laxatives are used to induce a bowel action and avoid constipation. They may overstimulate the muscles and lining of the bowel leading to irritation, spasm and in the long-term dilation (enlargement), and permanent damage of the colon. For this reason they should not be used on a regular basis.

Strong laxative herbs (cathartics) that should only be used occasionally for severe constipation, are senna and cascara. Conventional laxatives are things like phenolphthalein and dioctyl sodium sulphosuccinate, and although they work swiftly they can cause diarrhoea and cramping.

"Osmotic" laxatives such as magnesium sulphate and lactulose are a much safer alternative to cathartics and I prefer to use them in cases of severe occasional constipation. Osmotic laxatives draw water into the colon and make the bowel actions soft and watery. They do not generally irritate the bowels.

Suppositories and enemas are very effective for sudden severe constipation of the lower bowel. Some bowel therapists add herbs such as catnip or coffee to enemas to improve their cleansing effect.

Some people find that colonic irrigations are very beneficial in removing waste products from the bowel, and in experienced hands this is safe to do. However I would not encourage people to overly rely on enemas or colonic irrigations because regular bowel actions can be achieved through a high fibre diet and plenty of water and regular exercise. Enemas and/or colonic irrigations should not be performed in cases of inflammatory bowel disease, severe diverticulitis, or where there is a structural defect of the bowel. This is to avoid mechanical damage to the bowel in these cases.

Megacolon

In those who suffer with an enlarged bowel where there is dilation of the colon and extra (redundant) loops of bowel, the diagnosis of Megacolon can be made. This can be congenital or due to poor diet and laxative abuse. Where there is a very large amount of extra bowel, there may be huge redundant loops that trap food, which stagnates and putrefies inside them. This is a mechanical problem and causes abdominal bloating, swelling, flatulence and pain. The constipation produced is severe and it may be over a week before a bowel action eventuates. Understandably this is not helped even with strong laxatives. In this situation regular enemas and/ or colonic irrigation are essential. A special X ray called a Barium Enema *(see page 159)* is able to diagnose Megacolon with extra loops of unwanted bowel. In extreme cases the extra loops of bowel become huge and great help is achieved by surgically removing them in expert hands.

There are many fibre and herbal powders on the market that can increase the bulk of the faeces and reduce constipation. These are safe to use in the long term and confer general health benefits.

The best formula that I have found so far is called Fibretone and contains the following:

Soy bran	Carob powder	Carrot powder
Flaxseed (linseed) powder	Rice bran powder	Broccoli powder
Pectin	Guar gum	Spinach powder
Ginger root	Peppermint oil	Tomato powder
Slippery Elm powder	Beetroot powder	

Dosage of Fibretone is 2 tablespoons daily on cereal or in juice. Fibretone also contains useful nutritional substances for improving wellbeing. In this regard, it can be compared to the excellent nutritional powder, known as The Missing Link.

Fibretone is suitable for all types of constipation as it acts like an "intestinal broom," sweeping the walls of the colon clean, and so removing layers of encrusted and dried faecal matter. Make sure that you drink plenty of pure water (2 to 3 litres daily) to help this powder do its work.

It contains only soothing fibres and herbs and is effective for irritable bowel syndrome, abdominal bloating and chronic constipation. It can also reduce bowel toxicity caused by faecal stagnation, parasites and inflammation. Fibretone is also suitable for those who are allergic to gluten (found in wheat, oat, barley brans) or psyllium. Psyllium husks are a common ingredient in many bowel fibre powders and indeed can be very effective in constipation. However over a long period of time it is not uncommon for allergy to psyllium to occur, which may aggravate irritable bowel syndrome and cause itching and hay fever.

I include some letters from people who have used fibre powders:

Dear Health Advisory Service,
   I have been using a fibre powder for 10 weeks and I have noticed dramatic changes in my body. I had been a sufferer of abdominal bloating for 20 years and was most distressed to see my waistline getting larger every year. The bloating was much worse after eating and before my periods were due. I was unable to look nice in belts and my jeans would not fit which made me very depressed. No matter what I tried to wear I looked awful and like a "middle aged frump." I have always been constipated with small hard stools that would not come out easily. Since using the powder my bowel actions have changed completely so that I now go three times every day always at the same time. The bowel actions are larger and much longer, sometimes being over 12 inches long! My stomach has gradually gone down and I am now able to look feminine and slim in fashionable clothes. I am so happy to think that I have found a natural solution, although I wished I had understood my problem years ago to avoid all the suffering.

Dear Dr. Cabot
   I am a farmer who works with cattle and sheep and eat quite a lot of meat. I have been constipated for over 10 years and also suffered with irritable moods, haemorrhoids and itching around the anus. My wife finally got sick of my complaints and put me on Fibretone powder. For the first 8 days it did not change much, but on the 9th day I had a huge bowel action that was 2 feet long and very offensive in smell. When I examined it I saw hundreds of small worms wriggling around in it and two long ones as well. I was disgusted and told my doctor who tested my bowel actions and found several varieties of parasites. I have continued with the powder for 9 months with very good results and now have 2 largish bowel actions daily without straining. The itch and bad moods have gone and I have lost 23 kilograms in weight. I also take raw garlic daily and have no further signs of parasites.

Inflammatory Bowel Disease

This refers mainly to two chronic diseases that cause inflammation of the intestines: Ulcerative Colitis (UC) and Crohn's Disease (CD). Although UC and CD are different diseases they often cause similar symptoms. The severity of these diseases varies widely between individuals, with some having only mild symptoms whereas others have severe and disabling symptoms. Many researchers believe that inflammatory bowel disease is the result of an inherited predisposition that is triggered by an environmental agent (such as infection, food allergy, toxins or stress). It is not contagious. There does not appear to be a direct predictable pattern of inheritance, and around 15 to 20% of patients with inflammatory bowel disease (IBD) have immediate family members with IBD.

Ulcerative Colitis (UC)

Ulcerative colitis (UC) is an inflammatory disease of the large intestine, and causes inflammation and ulceration of the inner lining (mucosa) of the colon and rectum. Inflammation of the rectum is called proctitis. Inflammation of the sigmoid colon (situated just above the rectum) is called sigmoiditis. Inflammation of the entire colon is called pan-colitis. UC is autoimmune in origin, however it can flare up after emotional stress, food allergies and viral and bacterial infections. It is important to try and maintain a healthy population of microorganisms in the intestines to reduce infection of the inflamed bowel lining. For information on this *see page 105*. In UC the bowel lining becomes ulcerated releasing blood, mucous and pus.

Inflammation of the bowel lining causes the colon to empty too frequently, resulting in diarrhoea (sometimes explosive), cramping and flatulence. Bleeding from the rectum can occur and there may be up to 10 to 20 bowel actions containing blood and mucous daily. Weight loss, weakness, fever and dehydration often occurs during acute attacks.

Abscesses may form in the wall of the colon, which release infected pus into the colon. The colon may become very dilated and inflamed, which is a medical emergency known as toxic megacolon. Toxic megacolon occurs when inflammation spreads from the mucous lining through the remaining layers of the colon. The colon becomes paralysed which causes it to swell so much that it can eventually burst. This is known as a bowel perforation, which is a medical emergency often requiring surgery. The overuse of certain drugs, particularly opiate painkillers and antispasmodics may increase the risk of toxic megacolon. This is why drugs should be used with great care in both UC and CD.

UC begins most frequently in the age group 20 to 30, although older people and children occasionally develop this disease. A specialist gastroenterologist will carry out investigations such as barium enema X ray, and direct visualisation of the bowel lining using a fibre optic telescope.

Treatment of Ulcerative Colitis

The diet will have to be adjusted according to the severity of symptoms but needs to be high in easily absorbed forms of protein and carbohydrates. Protein powders made from whey, egg white and/or soy can be very helpful when solid foods can not be tolerated. High fibre foods may not be tolerated and indeed may aggravate the diarrhoea. In this situation raw vegetable and fruit juices made freshly with a juice-extracting machine and diluted with water can provide essential antioxidants, enzymes and healing phytonutrients. Dilute the juice so that you have 2 parts pure water to one part juice and drink 200 mls (7oz) every one to two hours. Selenium yeast powders can also be mixed into these diluted juices which provides easily absorbed forms of selenium and other antioxidants. These nutrients are essential to heal the ulcerated bowel lining. During acute flare-ups of the UC, avoid high fibre cereals, seeds and nuts and puree your fruits and vegetables after cooking them lightly. Eat only small frequent meals.

Food preparation takes longer for those with inflammatory bowel disease because it is much better to eat your fruits and vegetables finely chopped or grated after they have been washed thoroughly. All seeds and nuts should be finely ground in a coffee grinder or food processor.

It is important to avoid foods that may trigger attacks and everyone is different here. However I advise you to avoid dairy products, fried foods, sweet fizzy drinks and all preserved foods. If enjoyed, red meat can be eaten but should be very fresh and lean, very well cooked and eaten in small amounts only. Supplements of the fat-soluble vitamins, namely vitamins A, E, D and K should be taken regularly. Cod liver oil is a good source of these vitamins. If anaemia is present from the blood loss, tablets of organic iron, folic acid and vitamin B 12 injections are required.

Drug treatment is effective for the relief of acute symptoms in 70 - 80% of patients, and consists of antibiotics (sulfasalazine), antispasmodics and steroids. Often with the use of nutritional medicine, doses of steroid drugs can be minimised and confined to much shorter time periods. The minerals magnesium and potassium will need to be replaced because diarrhoea depletes these minerals. Surgery becomes necessary in severe cases where intestinal perforation or obstruction has occurred.

Long term regular follow up is essential, because for patients who have had UC for over 10 years, the risk of colon cancer is increased. Patients who have both UC and the liver disease Sclerosing Cholangitis , *see page 87*, may be at an even higher risk of colon cancer. These people should be screened with extra vigilance.

Crohn's Disease (CD)

Crohn's Disease (CD) is a severe inflammatory reaction that can affect any portion of the gastrointestinal tract from the oesophagus to the anus. It most commonly attacks the last part of the small intestine where it joins the colon in the ileocaecal area. Crohn's Disease is sometimes called ileitis, which refers to inflammation of the last part of the small intestine (ileum). In CD the inflammation of the bowel can be so deep that all layers of the bowel are affected. Eventually scarring may cause narrowing of the intestinal wall.

Symptoms of CD can include abdominal pain, anaemia, fatigue, flatulence, rectal bleeding, watery and bloody bowel actions, chronic diarrhoea, loud intestinal noises (borborygmus), fever, weight loss, loss of appetite, nausea and fissures in the anal area. Abdominal X ray reveals a thickened scarred and narrowed intestinal wall. The stools will test positive for blood and pus. Barium enema X ray shows lesions in the ileum. The specialist will have to assess severity by direct visualisation using a fibre optic telescope passed up through the rectum. This is called proctosigmoidoscopy and colonoscopy. A gastroscopy may also be required.

Treatment of Crohn's Disease (CD)

The diet must be adjusted according to the severity of the symptoms. The absorption of nutrients from the inflamed bowel lining may be poor, and it is usual to require a diet high in easily absorbed forms of protein and carbohydrates. Small frequent meals are better tolerated. The diet should also be low in animal fats. Dairy products should be avoided completely. **Ref 17**. When the bowel is inflamed high fibre foods are not tolerated well and many foods such as fruits and vegetables must be pureed in a blender.

British researchers have discovered that two-thirds of patients with CD, harbour in their intestine bacteria strikingly similar to the bacteria that causes Johne's disease in cattle. They also found this bacteria in pasteurised cows milk and they have found it to be very resilient to destruction, surviving in manure, soil and waterways.

Supplements of potassium and magnesium are needed after attacks of diarrhoea. Avoid laxatives and aspirin.

If the ileum is diseased be aware that vitamin B 12 deficiency may occur, and injections of vitamin B 12 should be given every 6 to 8 weeks. Deficiencies of fat-soluble vitamins may also occur which will reduce the ability of the bowel to heal and resist inflammation. For this reason it is wise to take supplements of the fat-soluble vitamins, namely vitamins A, D, E and K. These can be taken individually and are also present in cod liver oil and dark green and orange coloured vegetable and fruit juices. If you do not like the taste of cod liver oil, this is easily overcome by using capsules of cod liver oil, which can be taken just before meals. Take 2 capsules before every meal. It is not uncommon to find that people with CD have problems digesting and absorbing nutrients from food. Taking digestive enzymes with every meal can help this.

Drugs are required for acute attacks and consist of antibiotics (such as sulfasalazine, Azulfadine, flagyl), anti-spasmodics and steroids.

During a severe attack hospitalisation with intravenous hydration, intravenous steroids, total parenteral nutrition (nutrients given intravenously), and transfusions of packed red blood cells is often life saving. If the disease is not controlled properly complications such as intestinal obstruction, severe haemorrhaging, abscesses, infection, fistulas, malnutrition, perforation of the bowel, and toxic swelling of the entire colon (toxic megacolon) may supervene.

There may be a slightly higher risk of cancer of the small intestine or anus, and the lymphatic system (lymphoma) in suffers of CD. In those with longstanding (> 8 years) inflammatory disease of the colon, which involves more than the rectum and sigmoid colon, wether it be due to UC or CD, it is generally agreed by the experts that a regular screening colonoscopy should be done. This is to look for warning or early signs of cancer. If precancerous lesions are found most experts recommend removal of the colon (colectomy).

To reduce the risk of cancerous lesions evolving it is important to follow the basic principles of the Liver Cleansing Diet, *see pages 20 to 27.* It is also essential to supplement with the antioxidants selenium, vitamin C, vitamin E and vitamin A. These antioxidants have been proven to exert a protective effect against many types of cancers, including bowel cancer. Another excellent source of these antioxidants is raw vegetable juices such as carrot, beetroot, celery, apple, spinach, broccoli, cabbage, and any dark green leafy vegetables. These must be made freshly every day with a juice extractor. These juices are high in carotenoids including betacarotene (precursor to vitamin A) and other powerful anti-cancer phytonutrients.

Lactobacillus-acidophilus in the form of powder (must be refrigerated), or soy yoghurt with high culture counts should be used regularly in those with IBD.

Irritable Bowel Syndrome

This common problem has been known in the past by several names such as "spastic colon" or "nervous bowel". Irritable Bowel Syndrome (IBS) means an irritability of the bowel and this can affect any area of the digestive tract. A syndrome is a group of symptoms and signs that occur together and produce a typical pattern of a specific disorder.

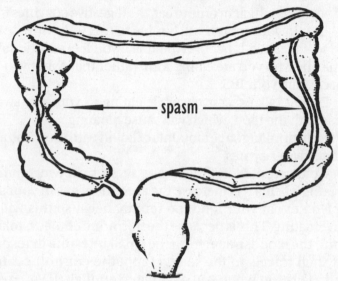

Spastic Colon

Classic symptoms of IBS are:

Abdominal pain- may vary from aching, dull, pressure, cramping, burning or sharp. The pains are usually intermittent and may disappear for long periods of time.

Altered pattern of the bowel actions - constipation, diarrhoea, or constipation alternating with diarrhoea.

Belching, bloating, nausea, reduced appetite and excessive gas.

The exact cause of IBS is unknown and is likely to be due to several factors operating together. To understand these factors, see causes of Bowel Dysfunction *on page104.*

In all sufferers the end result is a disordered rhythm in the muscles of the gastrointestinal tract. Normal intestinal contractions are called peristalsis, and consist of "segmental contractions" and "propulsive contractions". Segmental contractions churn and mix intestinal contents while propulsive contractions move the intestinal contents forwards on their way to the rectum for expulsion. Exaggerated segmental contractions may cause cramps, bloating and constipation. The forward movement of intestinal contents decreases and the bowel actions become harder and more compressed. This makes them hard to pass.

If the propulsive contractions are exaggerated, explosive watery diarrhoea may occur. This may cause an urgent desire to defecate, which can be very stressful, if a toilet is unavailable.

Treatment of Irritable Bowel Syndrome

• Set aside enough time to eat, and eat in a relaxed atmosphere. Think pleasant positive thoughts while eating and chew your food thoroughly. If you take sufficient time to eat, the digestive enzymes from the salivary glands in your mouth will be able to mix well with the food.

• Do not eat with people who make you feel emotionally disturbed. It may be who you are eating with, rather than what you are eating, that is causing your IBS.

• Do not talk excessively while eating as you may swallow excessive gas with the food, which will cause bloating.

• Avoid drinking large amounts of liquid with the meal, as this will dilute digestive enzymes.

• Avoid carbonated (fizzy) beverages or chewing gum or mints after eating, as this will increase the amount of gas in your stomach.

• Do not eat your food too rapidly because this will tend to cause overeating. This is because the hormone cholecystokinin is released into the bloodstream from the small intestine in response to a meal. It then travels to the satiety (appetite control) centre in the brain and tells you when you have eaten enough. If you rush down (gulp) your food there is insufficient time for the cholecystokinin hormone to switch off your hunger and you will probably overeat. It is far better to be a gourmet than a gourmand, and really experience the delicate flavours in every mouthful of your food.

• Avoid caffeine containing beverages, nicotine and a regular intake of alcohol.

• Follow the principles of the Liver Cleansing Diet found on *pages 20 to 27*. You may have to change your taste buds a little, however they will become accustomed to new flavours. If you have been eating lots of fat, salt and sugar you will need to reduce these things. One helpful way to consider salt, fat and sugar is as "flavour enhancers" rather than as foods. Their use can be minimised if you learn to use fresh herbs and spices to enhance food flavours. Cold pressed olive oil and other vegetable and seed oils can be added to hot vegetables rather than butter or margarine, and this will allow you to feel full and satisfied after the meal.

One of my patients had been a very obese woman or as she said a "yo-yo dieter." She told me that she had lost more than six hundred pounds in weight over the last 20 years and put more than that back on! She finally understood the importance of the liver in fat metabolism after reading my book, which allowed her to understand that "oils ain't oils." She started to replace heavy and damaged fats like butter, margarine and fatty meats with fish, lean veal and cold pressed oils. She told me that she used to make mashed potato with heaps of butter and salt, whereas now she cooks the potatoes and sprinkles them with olive oil. She will also add condiments to flavour the potatoes such as fresh garlic, chilli, coriander, healthy tomato or pesto sauces. She is able to feel satisfied after these foods because she is not on a low fat diet. Rather she is on the right fat diet, which is why she is now successful in keeping her weight and IBS under control.

Foods that may worsen IBS:

• Preserved and processed foods containing artificial colourings, preservatives or flavourings and gluten containing foods (wheat, rye, barley and oats), and dairy products.

• Some IBS sufferers are intolerant to the sugar found in milk, which is called lactose. Lactose intolerance results from a deficiency of the intestinal enzyme called lactase. Lactase is required to break down lactose into the simple sugars, glucose and galactose. Lactose intolerance is more common in Asian people and also becomes more frequent with age and after intestinal infections. If you are lactose intolerant but cannot live without dairy products it is possible to obtain cows milk that is processed to be lactose free. It is also possible to obtain tablets or drops containing the lactase enzyme, which can be taken with meals containing dairy products.

• Artificial sweeteners such as sorbitol or aspartame, and monosodium glutamate (MSG) can upset the bowels.

• Another thing that can trigger the symptoms of IBS is fructose (fruit sugar), which is found in all fruits and is used as a sweetener in some soft drinks. If you are intolerant to fructose (fruit sugar) you may find that juices of fruits and/or vegetables cause symptoms of IBS. This is because the juices concentrate the fructose. In this case you can dilute the juices with water, (2 parts water to 1 part juice is a good starting point) or rely on eating the whole fruits and vegetables. The extra fibre from the whole vegetable or fruit is more beneficial than pure juices in sufferers of IBS.

• Certain vegetables (such as cruciferous vegetables, garlic or onions) may give you unpleasant gas and bloating. This can be avoided by lightly cooking them and then blending them in a food processor or turning them into an Italian vegetable soup (minestrone).

If you suspect food intolerances to be causing your IBS, keep a food diary, which lists the foods you ate that day and the digestive symptoms experienced afterwards. Do this for 6 weeks and then go back over it and you may find some telltale patterns.

Check the Fibre Content of your Diet

Your diet should be providing 30 to 40 grams of fibre every day. If your diet is currently low in fibre you should increase your daily fibre intake gradually to allow your intestines to adjust. Otherwise you may suffer with bloating and excessive gas.

By gradually increasing dietary fibre you will over come many of the symptoms of irritable bowel syndrome. A high fibre intake has also been proven to reduce your chances of bowel cancer.

To help you increase fibre intake here is a list of high-fibre foods

Food	Dietary Fibre (grams)
Vegetables	
Asparagus, 1 cup	3.1
Beans, 1 cup pinto	5.3
Beans, 1 cup green	2.1
Beans, 1 cup kidney	5.8
Beetroot, 1 cup	2.5
Broccoli, 1 cup	3.0
Brussels sprouts, 1 cup	2.8
Cabbage, 1 cup	2.8
Cauliflower, 1 cup	1.8
Lettuce, 1 cup	0.5
Onion, 1 cup	2.1
Carrots, 1 cup	3.0
Peas, 1 cup	5.0
Potato, 1 medium baked	3.0
Spinach, 1 cup cooked	5.7
Tomatoes, 1 medium	1.4
Turnips, 2/3 cup	2.0
Sweet corn,1/2 cup	4.7
Zucchini, 1 cup	2.7
Fruits	
Apple, 1 medium	2.8
Banana, 1 medium	1.8
Berries, 1 cup	2.0
Cherries, 16 large	1.0
Figs, 2 dried	6.4
Grapes, 15	2.0
Orange, 1 medium	3.2
Peach, 1 medium	2.2
Pineapple, 1/3 cup	0.5

Food	Dietary Fibre (grams)
Fruits	
Plums, 2 small	1.5
Prunes, 6 medium	2.0
Strawberries, 12 medium	2.0
Grains/Cereals/Nuts	
Corn flakes, 1 cup	2.0
Wheat bran, 1 cup	2.5
Shredded wheat, 1 wafer	2.7
Rice, (brown) cooked, 1/2 cup	2.4
Rice, (white) cooked, 1 cup	0.1
Brazil nuts, 1/3 cup	2.9
Peanuts, 1 cup	6.6
Sunflower seeds, 1 cup	8.0
Bread	
Wholegrain, (wheat) 1 slice	1.4
White bread, 1 slice	0.5
Rye bread, 1 slice	1.0

Dietary fibre is found in two different forms:

1. **Soluble** fibre which dissolves in water such as mucilages, gums and pectins.
2. **Insoluble** fibre which does not dissolve in water such as cellulose, most hemicelluloses and lignans.

Vegetables, fruits and grains contain a mixture of these two types of fibre. Wheat bran consists of mainly insoluble fibres whereas oat bran contains mainly soluble fibre. In the colon, fibre is acted upon by friendly bacteria which causes fermentation of the fibrous food remnants in the colon. This helps to make the stools soft, moist and larger, which means they are easier to pass. They also travel along the large bowel easily without requiring undue contractions from the bowel. Beans contain gums, which are a good source of water-soluble fibres. Sweetcorn contains a mixture of fibres and is an excellent food for those wanting to improve their bowel patterns. Raw fruits and vegetables are an excellent cleansing source of both types of fibre.

I have had several patients who have complained of excessive gas and bloating after increasing their intake of beans, seeds and raw vegetables. Remember to increase these things very gradually, using only small amounts to begin with. You can also take one tablespoon of apple cider vinegar mixed in water and sip it slowly during the meal. Another tip that often works is to use digestive enzyme tablets or powders during the meal.

Many suffers of IBS do not drink enough water which will increase symptoms of constipation and flatulence. I have found that increasing water intake to at least 2 litres daily will overcome many of the symptoms of IBS. Drink this water in between meals.

For very acute and severe attacks of IBS that can be precipitated by stress or really letting go of your diet, medication may be needed. This may require the use of drugs to stop spasm in the muscles of the bowel (antispasmodics), laxatives for severe constipation or drugs to stop diarrhoea. You should see your doctor for these things and self-medication is not advisable.

Prolapsed Colon

The transverse colon goes from the right side to the left side of the body and is made of soft muscular tissue. If the transverse colon becomes overloaded with faeces the force of gravity will cause it to droop down or prolapse into the lower abdominal and pelvic cavities. *See diagram below*

A prolapsed transverse colon will put pressure on the lower abdominal and pelvic organs. Weakness of the abdominal muscles, and excessive fat inside the abdominal cavity and in the abdominal wall, will further increase the downward forces upon the transverse colon. The prolapsed transverse colon will press onto the bladder and uterus and may cause urinary frequency and pelvic congestion. In men this may lead to congestion of the prostate gland causing frequency of urination. The chronically prolapsed transverse colon may become very enlarged and twisted, producing extra loops of swollen colon which is known as redundant bowel. Redundant bowel is useless bowel and acts like a

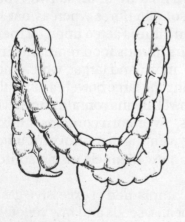

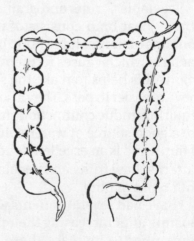

Prolapsed Colon

Healthy Colon

stagnant reservoir for fermentation and putrefaction of faeces. This leads to an increase in unfavourable bacteria in the bowel and reabsorption of toxins from the bowel into the blood stream, which is carried back to the liver. This process is known as autointoxication and can cause severe flatulence and chronic ill health.

To reduce this problem it is vital to follow a regular exercise program including abdominal exercises, brisk walking and swimming. Regular Yoga can be especially helpful for prolapsed colon. Massage of the abdominal area in the direction of the movement of the faeces can be very helpful if done regularly. Avoidance of constipation is essential, *see page 114.*

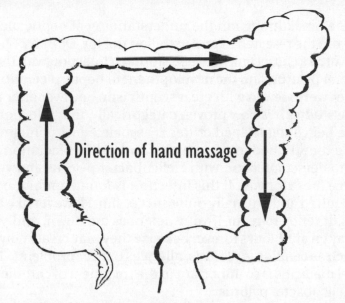

Direction of hand massage

Massage of abdomen to reduce constipation

Peptic Ulcers

These types of ulcers refer to those found in the stomach (gastric ulcers), or first section of the small intestine (duodenal ulcers). These ulcers look like raw areas of erosion and can be small or large, singular or multiple, and deep or superficial, *see diagram on page 129.*

I well remember when I worked in a missionary hospital in the Himalayan foothills during the mid 1980's, that a very large number of young to middle aged Indian males came to the hospital with acute rupture of peptic ulcers. This is a life-threatening emergency and needless to say a good percentage of them perished from the septicaemia and peritonitis that ensued after rupture. I finally discovered that the cause was the home made alcoholic brew that was part of their culture in that area. This combined with a marginal diet and smoking "Indian Bidi" cigarettes had made them vulnerable to ulceration of the stomach and duodenum.

Symptoms of peptic ulcers can range from "hunger pains" to an intense burning pain in the upper abdomen that will make you double up in agony. This pain is usually worse at night and when the stomach is empty. Stress can also bring on an attack. Eating food and drinking milk will often temporarily deaden the pain.

Factors that can cause or exacerbate peptic ulcers are stress, poor diet, missing meals, nutritional deficiencies, smoking, alcohol excess, analgesic drugs and anti-inflammatory drugs (both non-steroidal and steroidal varieties).

In 1982 a breakthrough in the understanding of peptic ulcer disease resulted from the research of an Australian doctor, Dr Barry Marshall. He had discovered a causal link between stomach infection with the bacteria, Helicobacter pylorus, and the development of peptic ulceration. Initially his theories were viewed with great scepticism, however after numerous worldwide studies it is now proven categorically, that infection with this nasty little helicopter shaped critter is associated with inflammation of the stomach and duodenum, which can lead to ulceration. Tests are available to detect infection with Helicobacter pylorus and your doctor can arrange these for you. If this infection is found antibiotic treatment may be required and is usually quite successful. However like all chronic infections, it tends to recur if your defences are down, and you do not want to stay on antibiotics forever because they may create new problems for you such as candida, dysbiosis, allergies or liver problems. This is why nutritional medicine is so important in the treatment of chronic infections such as Helicobacter pylorus.

The diet should consist of small frequent meals that contain plenty of vegetables, fruits, grains and legumes. During acute attacks it may be more comfortable to eat only home made soups (vegetable and/or chicken), steamed vegetables and fish and rice.

"Smoothies" made with soymilk, banana, papaya and raw egg are soothing and healing and small amounts can be drunk regularly throughout the day. Bananas contain phospholipids that are surface active and needed to maintain the protective layer on the stomach mucosa. Raw vegetable juices containing carrot, celery, apple and beetroot are beneficial for their healing and soothing properties. Raw cabbage juice has been traditionally used to heal ulcers. It is effective, despite its taste, because it contains "substance U" which has powerful ulcer healing properties. Cabbage is also high in the liver amino acid glutamine, which stimulates mucin synthesis to enhance mucosal healing. The cabbage juice can be mixed with the other juices mentioned here to improve its flavour.

Generally speaking the diet should be along the lines of the Liver Cleansing Diet found on *pages 20 to 27* of this book.

Peptic Ulcer

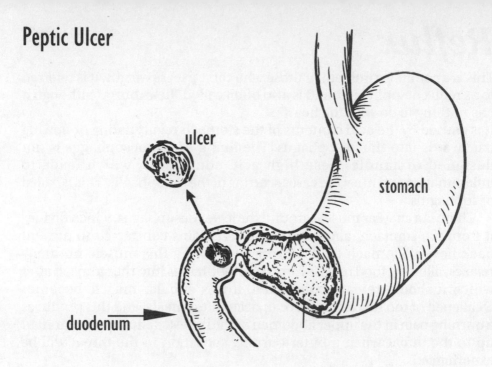

Natural Remedies for Peptic Ulcers

• Slippery Elm powder stirred into oat or rice milk or juices can be used as desired, as it is free of side effects.
• Vitamins A and E, and the minerals Zinc and Selenium will speed healing and improve the health of the mucosal lining.
• Essential fatty acid supplements such as flaxseed oil and cod liver oil will strengthen the mucosal membranes.
• Herbal teas such as chamomile, arrowroot, marshmallow, liquorice and golden seal are soothing and healing. These can be sweetened with a little honey (not sugar) if desired, and are preferable to coffee and tea (especially strong tea) if you have peptic ulcers.

If infection with the stomach bacteria Helicobacter pylorus is a chronic problem, take Olive Leaf capsules, using a 500 mg capsule at the beginning of every meal. Olive leaf contains oleuropein, which can fight unwanted intestinal bacteria and parasites. It is safe to take Olive leaf extract long term and it does not interact with any drugs that you may be taking.

Reflux

This is a common problem in those who carry excess weight. It is referred to as reflux oesophagitis, and is also often called "heartburn," although it has nothing to do with the heart.

It is caused by the acid contents of the stomach regurgitating or flowing backwards into the oesophagus. The lining of the oesophagus is not designed to handle these high acid conditions, which leads to inflammation and in severe cases scarring of the oesophagus. This is called oesophagitis.

There is a circular muscle around the lower oesophagus, which divides it from the stomach, and this normally remains contracted to prevent back flow of stomach acid. During swallowing this muscle normally relaxes, allowing food to pass from the oesophagus into the stomach after which it should remain contracted. If this circular muscle becomes weakened or too relaxed, reflux can occur after meals, and this produces a burning pain in the upper abdomen or mid chest. Reflux can occur right up to the throat when a bitter burning sensation in the throat will be experienced.

In some people with reflux there is also a hernia (protrusion) of the upper part of the stomach through the diaphragm into the lower chest. This is called a hiatus hernia and is more common with age and in those who are overweight. A hiatus hernia will often disturb the function of the circular muscle around the lower oesophagus. This increases reflux and heartburn symptoms. These symptoms are much worse after eating a large meal and while bending over.

If you suffer with long standing oesophageal reflux it is important to see your gastroenterologist regularly, because prolonged exposure of the fragile oesophageal mucosa to acid can result in an increased risk of oesophageal cancer and severe scarring and stricture formation. The passage inside the oesophagus can become so narrowed that difficulty swallowing normal amounts and types of food will result, and severe pain may occur. Surgery to enlarge the lower oesophagus may then become necessary.

In severe cases of reflux oesophagitis, medications to block stomach acid production should be taken if natural therapies fail. These are very effective and generally well tolerated. Examples of these drugs are cimetidine, famotidine, nizatidine, rantidine and omeprazole.

To reduce reflux these techniques often work well.

- If overweight it is important to reduce your weight with regular exercise and correct diet.
- Meals should be small and frequent as large meals increase pressure inside the stomach.

- Do not drink with meals and confine your fluid intake to between meals.
- Do not eat food during the 3 hours before retiring to bed and drink alkaline beverages during this time such as herbal teas, aloe vera juice, and water or celery juice.
- Elevate the top of your bed by 6 to 8 inches by placing blocks under the head of the bed. Avoid tight fitting clothes around the middle and do not bend over after meals.
- Avoid coffee, alcohol, cigarettes, fatty foods, and fried foods, preserved foods and vinegar. Some people find that spicy food such as chilli or curry will aggravate symptoms.

Natural Supplements to reduce reflux:

- Magnesium Complete- 1 tablet twice daily, at the beginning of meals, to help the oesophageal muscle.
- Slippery elm powder mixed in soy milk, water or juice can reduce acidity; take it after or in between meals.
- Vitamin E will reduce scarring of the oesophagus.
- Vitamin A will promote healing of the mucous membranes.
- Soothing herbal teas are chamomile, marshmallow, alfalfa, meadowsweet, golden seal, and liquorice root. You can add a little honey to sweeten if desired.

If you get an acute attack of heartburn it is acceptable to use an antacid preparation for quick relief. Avoid aluminium containing antacids and use potassium or sodium bicarbonate, magnesium carbonate or hydroxide instead.

Coeliac Disease

Coeliac disease is due to a sensitivity to gluten, which is a compound found in the grains wheat, barley, rye and oats. The term "sensitivity" is not the same as "allergy," and implies a much more severe reaction in the body.

The gluten damages the cells lining the small intestine, and the mucosal surface becomes flat, losing the normal folds known as villi. These damaged mucosal cells are unable to absorb nutrients from the food and severe nutritional deficiencies eventually occur.

Coeliac disease is common in Europe with an incidence in the UK of 1 in 2000, and in Ireland of 1 in 300. It occurs worldwide but is rare in the indigenous population of Africa. The cause is often hereditary, however the exact mode of inheritance is not clear. The disease can begin at any age and in children, it appears after weaning them onto gluten containing foods. In adults it usually begins in the third and fourth decade, and is more common in females.

The symptoms are usually very gradual in onset and may start with only fatigue. Common intestinal symptoms include abdominal discomfort, bloating, diarrhoea, and weight loss. There is difficulty in absorbing fat from the food. This makes the bowel actions large, pale and fatty so that they tend to float on top of the water and are difficult to flush down the toilet. Mouth ulcers and dermatitis around the corners of the mouth are common. People with coeliac disease have a higher incidence of allergies and autoimmune diseases (including thyroid, diabetes, inflammatory bowel disease and chronic liver disease).

Many of the symptoms of coeliac disease are similar to those of irritable bowel syndrome (IBS), so if symptoms do not abate with treatment for IBS, it is important to think of excluding coeliac disease.

A blood test is available to detect this abnormal sensitivity to gluten. It is called the antigliaden antibody test. This test is more accurate in children, and in adults can give false results - either false positives or false negatives. The only categorical way to make an accurate diagnosis of coeliac disease is by removing a tiny piece of the mucosal lining of the upper small intestine for examination under a microscope. This is called a biopsy and is done through a fibre optic telescope passed through the mouth.

Thankfully this disease responds extremely well to dietary modification. If patients stick to a gluten free diet they generally remain very well, and the mucosal lining of the small intestine returns to normal. Normal absorption of nutrients is then possible, although it is important to check periodically for deficiencies of iron, folic acid, vitamin B 12 and fat-soluble vitamins (vitamins A, D, E and K). This is easily done with a blood test.

Because these patients are more likely to suffer with immune dysfunction I think it is wise for them to supplement their diets with Vitamins E, C and A and selenium. Essential fatty acid supplements such as flaxseed oil and cod liver oil are also worthwhile to strengthen the cell membranes in the cells lining the small intestines.

Gluten Free Diet

This involves the exclusion of wheat, rye, barley and oats. All foods containing gluten - whether it be obvious, (eg. bread, flour) or hidden (eg. most sausages, stock cubes) MUST BE AVOIDED.

Allowed Foods - Gluten-free (GF)

Gluten-free (GF) bread, GF pasta, GF biscuits & crackers, GF flour
Flour made from potato, soy, peas, and rice
Bran made only from rice, soy
GF cakes & biscuits

Rice, tapioca, arrowroot, maize, millet, sago, buckwheat, amaranth, quinoa and teff
Fresh or frozen poultry & meat
Fish fresh or frozen, or canned in oil
Eggs
Milk, butter, cream, oils
Vegetables plain, fresh or canned (including potatoes)
Fruit plain, fresh, frozen or canned & their juices
Nuts, legumes & seeds
Sugar, honey, jam, gelatine, rice syrup, boiled lollies
Herbs, spices, pepper, salt, mustard, vinegar

Forbidden Foods - Contain Gluten

Regular breads, crackers, biscuits, pasta
Regular flour, rye flour, barley flour
Bran from wheat, oats
Regular cakes and biscuits
Breakfast cereals containing wheat, oats, barley or rye
Semolina
Pies, pasties, most beefburgers, most sausages, many tinned meats
Meat or fish with breadcrumbs or batter, fish cakes,
Potato croquettes
Barley water
Most stock cubes and gravy mixes

This list is not exhaustive and there are other things that you may need to avoid. This is because it is not always possible to tell from food labels if a processed product is gluten-free.

The Coeliac Society produces complete lists of processed foods that are gluten free and if you would like more information contact the Coeliac Society in your state.

These are the postal addresses of the Coeliac Societies in Australia
P.O. Box 271, Wahroonga, NSW. 2076
P.O. Box 89, Holmesglen, VIC. 3148
P.O. Box 159, Launceston, TAS. 7250
P.O. Box 219, Mt. Lawley, WA. 6050
P.O. Box 530, Indooropilly, QLD 4068
106A Hampstead Rd. Broadview, SA. 5083

The Coeliac Society of South Australia can provide a good range of gluten free foods for everyday use and also for special occasions. They have a price list and do mail order all over Australia. They also publish several excellent gluten free recipe books.

Interesting Healthful Grains

Amaranth

This was the grain used traditionally by the Aztec Indians of North America. Amaranth is now becoming popular again amongst health conscious people. It is very high in protein and is a good source of complex carbohydrates. Amaranth is gluten free and can be used as a substitute for wheat in those with coeliac disease. It needs to be presoaked and cooked on a low heat to facilitate digestion. You can use it in casseroles and stews alone or combined with other grains.

Kamut

Kamut is another ancient grain originating from the Fertile Crescent thousands of years ago. It is a relative of modern Durham wheat and has a lovely nutty flavour. Kamut contains gluten and may not be tolerated by those with coeliac disease. It is very high in protein and fatty acids as well as the minerals magnesium and zinc and is more nutritious than regular wheat. You can use kamut in casseroles, stews, soups or salads. It is nice in a salad too. Simply cook it in boiling water for around 1 and 1/2 hours and then cool in a refrigerator. Mix it with a selection of chopped raw vegetables and add plain soy yoghurt and olive oil. You may season salad with any fresh herbs, paprika, curry powder or vegetable seasoning according to your taste.

Quinoa

Quinoa is another ancient grain and was traditionally used by the Incas. It is high in protein and can be used as a substitute for rice and wheat in many dishes. It is easy to digest and those with wheat allergies or irritable bowel syndrome find it of benefit. Quinoa is gluten free and is tolerated by those with coeliac disease. It is also good for those with intolerance to dairy products because it is very high in calcium.

Other grain substitutes for wheat and rice that you may like to try to give you more variety are spelt, teff, millet, buckwheat and yellow cornmeal. Spelt is a form of wheat and contains gluten. Teff and buckwheat are gluten free and should be tolerated by those with coeliac disease. Millet is gluten free and can be consumed by those with coeliac disease. Millet sometimes becomes contaminated with wheat and other sources of gluten during harvesting, storage and processing of mixed crops.

All of these grains are good sources of fibre, complex carbohydrates, protein and minerals. They are good bone building foods.

amaranth casserole   serves 4

1 cup	amaranth, cooked
1 cup	rice or millet,cooked
3 cloves	garlic
1 cup	carrots, sliced
1 cup	cabbage, chopped
1	zucchini, chopped
1 cup	capsicum chopped
1 cup	fresh tomatoes, chopped
425g (15oz)	whole tomatoes, tinned, chopped (keep juice)
4 tbsp	cold pressed olive oil
3 tbsp	fresh basil
2	shallots, chopped
2	brown onions, chopped

Sauté olive oil with garlic, shallots and onions.
Add all vegetables and saute for 4 minutes.
Add canned tomatoes and their juice, amaranth and rice (or millet).
Simmer for 10 minutes and season to taste with mineral salt, tamari, soy sauce or vegetable seasoning.
Make sure the vegetables are still crisp and do not overcook.

Haemorrhoids

Haemorrhoids are dilated and inflamed veins that occur in the lower rectum and anal area. They can be considered as varicose veins in the rectum. They may have blood clots inside them which make them hard and swollen. Symptoms can range from mild discomfort to extreme pain, making it impossible to sit down. They may cause anal itching, a mucous discharge and bleeding, with bright red blood seen in the toilet bowl and on the toilet paper after wiping. Haemorrhoids should always be assessed by a doctor to exclude more sinister causes of bleeding.

If possible try to control them with natural therapies and diet because surgery is often only temporarily effective. The surgical techniques most commonly used today are cryotherapy (freezing of the haemorrhoid), or placing rubber bands to strangle the haemorrhoids. These techniques are thankfully a far cry from the painful haemorrhoidectomy procedure of years gone by.

Haemorrhoids are more common in those who have a sluggish congested liver, chronic constipation, obesity and high alcohol intake.

To overcome Haemorrhoids try the following:
• Increase fibre in the diet by eating raw vegetables and fruits, bran, millet, buckwheat Fibretone and ground flaxseed (linseed).

- Drink plenty of water, herbal teas and vegetable juices.
- Take a good liver tonic in powder form, 2 tsp daily, in juice.
- Take vitamin E 1000 i.u. daily.
- Take vitamin C powder 2000 mg daily.
- Drink organic apple cider vinegar 2 tablespoons in a glass of water with half a teaspoon of honey daily.
- Eat buckwheat, and berry fruits (especially red and black coloured) as they are high in bioflavonoids, which strengthen blood vessel walls.
- Herbal teas of horse chestnut and nettle, and dandelion coffee.
- Local creams can be applied containing local anaesthetic/steroid combinations for short-term relief of acute severe haemorrhoids. For long term treatment use herbal creams/ointments containing the herbs witch hazel, calendula, golden seal or hypericum.
- Sit in a warm salt bath with 3 tablespoons of sea salt dissolved in the water. This will provide cleansing and soothing of the rectal area. If you are plagued with recurrent haemorrhoids, consider installing a bidet.
- Regular exercise and the avoidance of prolonged standing are important. Avoid straining during bowel movements. When haemorrhoids are present they often cause a full feeling or what is referred to as a sense of incomplete evacuation after a bowel action. This may cause you to strain and push to get the last bit of stool out, when in reality all the stool is gone. In this situation further straining will only push the haemorrhoids out, causing prolapse.
- Reduce stress as this can bring on a haemorrhoid attack. Magnesium Complete is a good remedy for stress induced haemorrhoids.

Diverticulosis & Diverticulitis

Diverticulosis refers to small blind pockets or pouches that form in the wall of the colon and are very common in people over 60 years of age. They may not cause any symptoms and may be discovered on a barium enema X ray.

These pouches form because of weak spots in the circular muscles of the colon. In those who do not consume enough dietary fibre, the colonic muscles must work much harder to propel undigested food along the colon to the rectum. These excessive contractions increase the pressure inside the colon leading to stretched and weakened areas in the bowel wall. The small pouches or diverticula then pop through or "blow out" in these weakened areas. Excessive use of strong laxatives in those with chronic constipation can also cause diverticula, because these drugs lead to excessive colonic contractions and high internal bowel pressures.

If there is no inflammation in the bowel pockets the condition is referred to as Diverticulosis. Diverticulosis may not produce any symptoms in some people whereas others will suffer with bloating, irregular bowel actions and some abdominal cramps.

Sometimes undigested food can become trapped inside these bowel pockets, and then bacteria start to work on it, causing

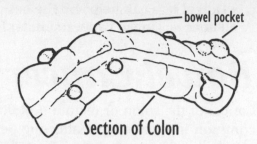

bowel pocket

Section of Colon

fermentation and putrefaction of the food particles. This can lead to foul smelling wind and abdominal swelling and cramps. Colonic irrigations and enemas may help but can only be used with caution under medical supervision.

If the bowel pocket becomes very inflamed and infected, the condition of Diverticulitis occurs which can be very serious. The bowel pocket may leak bacteria into the normally sterile abdominal cavity causing severe inflammation and even peritonitis. Symptoms of fever and severe abdominal pain and tenderness, particularly in the left lower abdomen may occur. This is treated with antibiotics, intravenous therapy and fasting. Rarely the diverticula may rupture, spilling infected food contents into the abdominal cavity and this may cause rectal bleeding.

Treatment of Diverticulosis

The diet needs to be modified in those with diverticulosis and there needs to be a gradual increase in dietary fibre. This will reduce the pressure inside the colon and improve bowel habits and symptoms.

• Do not eat foods containing small nuts and seeds (found in some breads, muesli and biscuits) as these small things can become trapped inside the bowel pockets. Seeds and nuts are very healthy and you may still enjoy them if you take the time to grind them into a fine powder in a coffee grinder or food processor. In this powder form they will not aggravate diverticulosis, and indeed should help the condition by boosting dietary fibre.

• Drink plenty of pure water in between your meals, as this will greatly reduce symptoms.

• Have small frequent meals with plenty of raw fruits and vegetables.

• You may need to spend extra time in food preparation to grind wholegrains and muesli, grate vegetables and finely cut fruits. Remove all pips and seeds lest they get stuck in the pockets.

• Use soy yoghurt and raw garlic (finely grated or juiced), and take supplements of lactobacillus acidophilus to reduce the chances of infection of the bowel pockets.

• If constipation does occur the safest laxatives to use in this condition are osmotic laxatives, such as Lactulose and magnesium sulphate.

- Herbal teas can help and the best ones are chamomile, dandelion, echinacea, ginger, peppermint, and yellow dock and aloe vera juice.

Bowel Cancer

Cancer of the colon or rectum (ColoRectal Cancer or CRC) is the most common internal cancer affecting people in the Western world, with around 1 in 20 persons being affected. CRC is second only to lung cancer in terms of mortality rates. The incidence of CRC in Australia is one of the highest in the world and is higher again in New Zealand.

Risk Factors for ColoRectal Cancer (CRC)

1. Genetic factors

These are important and there is a genetic predisposition to bowel polyps and CRC.

If a person has one first-degree relative with bowel polyps or CRC, their risk of CRC approximates to 1 in 8 over their lifetime. Bowel polyps are cauliflower-like growths that arise out of the mucosal lining of the bowel on a stalk. Spontaneous genetic mutations leading to cancer cells can also occur in bowel polyps in those with no family history of cancer.

2. Dietary Factors

Factors that increase CRC are a high fat, low fibre, high alcohol diet. A high fibre diet reduces the usual risk of CRC by a whopping 50%.

3. Inflammatory bowel diseases

Those with long-standing Ulcerative Colitis and Crohn's Disease are at higher risk of CRC.

Signs of Bowel Cancer

ColoRectal Cancer (CRC) typically does not produce any symptoms or signs in its early stages and has often been growing slowly for years before it is diagnosed. Unfortunately often there are no symptoms or signs at all until the late stages of cancer growth.

When symptoms and signs begin they may consist of bleeding from the rectum, a change in bowel patterns (constipation, diarrhoea, urgency), abdominal discomfort, iron deficiency anaemia or weight loss. If you have any bleeding from the bowels, a gastroenterologist who will visualise the bowel directly with a flexible telescope, must investigate this. This is called sigmoidoscopy or colonoscopy. X rays such as barium enemas are not sufficiently accurate to investigate the causes of bleeding from the bowels.

Sometimes the cancer may spread to other parts of the body before it produces any symptoms. A common site of spread is to the liver, and sometimes the bowel cancer is first detected when its satellite growths (metastases) cause enlargement of the liver and fluid in the abdomen.

Bowel Polyps

Some types of bowel polyps may undergo malignant changes, which is tantamount to early bowel cancer. From these small cancers, a large cancer can grow often silently and remain undetected for years. If the doctor discovers that you have polyps growing in the colon during a colonoscopy, they can be removed at this time using a procedure known as a polypectomy. They will then be tested for cancer cells. You will be advised to have regular colonoscopies done to check for recurrence.

If you are a person who keeps on developing polyps in the colon, it is advisable to use nutritional medicine with the aim of preventing more polyps, and also preventing cancerous changes in any new polyps that develop in between your regular colonoscopies. You should increase fibre in the diet, and consume plentiful amounts of raw vegetables and fruit. You will need to reduce your intake of red meat and avoid all dairy products and preserved meats. Make sure that everything you eat is fresh and try to source organically raised produce *(see page 287)*. Supplements of vitamin C, E and A, along with the mineral selenium, should be taken daily to reduce the risk of cancerous changes.

Early Detection of Bowel Cancer

The chances of survival after CRC are related to the stage at which it is discovered. Early detection and treatment give a much better outlook. For this reason it is vital to identify patients in the early stages of CRC who will probably have no symptoms, as well as those with bowel polyps which may become malignant.

This requires screening of the general population and surveillance of high-risk patients.

Screening of general population for Bowel Cancer:
- Ideally should start at age 50.
- Test stools for hidden blood (faecal occult blood test). This is done through your family doctor.
- If stools test positive for blood, see a gastroenterologist who will visualise the rectum and colon with a flexible fibre optic telescope (sigmoidoscopy to check lower bowel, or colonoscopy to check the entire colon and rectum).

Surveillance of high-risk individuals for Bowel Cancer:
- Ideally should start at age 40.
- Colonoscopy to find polyps or early cancer.
- If no polyps found, repeat colonoscopy every 3 to 5 years.

• If polyps found they must be removed and colonoscopy should be done more frequently until polyps stop recurring.

Prevention of Bowel Cancer

• Reduce your consumption of animal meat and animal fat.
• Reduce your consumption of preserved foods, especially preserved and smoked meats.
• Reduce your consumption of alcohol.
• Eat plenty of fibre, which is found in raw vegetables, raw fruits, wholegrain, bran, cereals, muesli, legumes, seeds and nuts.
• Ensure adequate antioxidants especially vitamins C, A, E, and selenium. I have met very few people with a perfect diet, and even if you do have one, in this day and age, you cannot guarantee that you will get all the antioxidants you need to reduce your risk of cancer.
• Follow the principles of the Liver Cleansing Diet found on *pages 20 to 27*. A healthy liver will protect your immune system from overload. A strong immune system is your greatest weapon against bowel cancer.

Nutritional Help for those with Liver and Bowel Cancer

• Easily digested foods such as vegetable and grain soups, pureed vegetables and raw vegetable juices. Suitable juices are beetroot, carrot, and celery, apple and wheat grass juice. These can be diluted with 50% water if desired. Drink around 300 - 500 mls (10 - 17oz)of this juice mixture daily. Protein powder food supplements from soy or whey are beneficial, and can be added to smoothies made with oat, rice or soymilk, soy yoghurt and banana.
• Eat fish at least three times a week such as sardines, salmon and tuna (canned varieties are acceptable).
• Try to eat a wide variety of green leafy vegetables, raw and lightly steamed. The cruciferous vegetables (broccoli, cauliflower, Brussels sprouts and cabbage) have proven anti-cancer properties.
• Evidence from Japan suggests that an organic compound of germanium has anti-cancer effects. It appears to stimulate interferon synthesis and immune function. Germanium is present in garlic, shiitake mushrooms and champignon mushrooms.
• Eat Brazil nuts and garlic because they contain selenium, which has anti-tumour effects.
• Digestive enzymes such as pancreatin should be taken with every meal. To enhance digestive enzymes eat foods that are rich in their own enzymes such as papaya, beetroot, sprouts, avocado, banana, mango and pineapple.
• Free range eggs can be eaten (one or two at a time) if desired because of their high content of liver friendly amino acids, and are a convenient form of complete protein.

- **Use** foods and supplements to boost the body's production of natural interferon. Interferon is produced by normal body cells to keep cancer cells and viruses under control. It regulates immune cells and their defensive capability, and is vitally important for cancer sufferers.

The following substances will help to boost your natural interferon production:

- Chlorophyll (found in dark green vegetables and wheat grass juice)
- Vitamin C with bioflavonoids, 1000mg with every meal.
- Sea vegetables (such as hijiki, kombu, wakame, kelp, agar, Irish moss, nori, dulse)
- Blue-green algae such as spirulina

Immune boosting herbs are:
St Mary's Thistle, Echinacea and Olive leaf extract.

The excellent book "Heal Cancer" by Dr. Ruth Cilento, and published by Hill of Content, is an invaluable dietary guide for those with cancer.

My Recovery From Bowel Cancer

by Trish Pemberton

It came out of the blue. I had always been healthy. One day when I stood up from the toilet I noticed a dark blood clot in the toilet bowl. I was puzzled. My first thought was 'maybe I've got haemorrhoids'. I didn't see this as a problem because there are treatments available to make haemorrhoids less painful, yet strangely, I didn't have any pain. I became concerned.

An ache in my heel had been a constant companion for more than a month. Massage didn't help. If I had known anything about Reflexology before I was diagnosed, I may have been aware of what was happening inside. Later I found out that that part of the heel relates to the large bowel. When I woke up after the surgery I no longer had the ache in my foot.

I went to the doctor who checked me by probing in my anus with a rubber gloved finger. This was uncomfortable but not painful. The blood from haemorrhoids is light she told me. My clot was dark, I didn't have haemorrhoids. She considered my case urgent and that day made an appointment for me to see a surgeon who specialises in the bowel area.

Everything happened so quickly I didn't have much time to think about what was going on in my body and what was going to happen. I went along for the ride as the doctors seemed to take over my life. I was in shock. I was so stunned that I didn't object to the suggested treatment.

Apart from the blood clot and ache in my foot, I had no other symptoms. There was no pain, no constipation or spurting. After I was diagnosed I was told by all and sundry, that I was too young in my early forties to have bowel cancer, especially as there is no family history of it.

The surgeon checked me using the same technique as the GP, but he probed further - quite painful. It proved that there was a mass close to the base of the large bowel. He arranged for me to see the doctor who performs colonoscopies. I was booked in the next week and was given instructions for the day before.

That day I was to take only fluids - jelly, soup, that sort of thing. From 3 pm I started to drink 3 litres of a dreadful mixture, Glycoprep, to prepare my bowel for the colonoscopy. It reacts with the bowel to clear it so that the bowel wall can be seen clearly during the process. About three hours later there was the first of many rushes to the toilet. These continued at more frequent intervals for a few hours.

The Colonoscopy

At the hospital, dressed in an open-backed, neck to knee gown, I was wheeled to the operating theatre and sedated. I woke up in a screened area. The doctor confirmed that the mass in my bowel was cancer.

I went back to the surgeon to arrange the operation. He showed me a photograph taken during the colonoscopy. Whereas the bowel is normally round like a tube and clear, I had less than an eighth of the space open. The remainder was tumour. I had to have it removed. I would need time in hospital and time to recover. It was like a bad dream.

The surgeon said that until he operated he would not know the extent of the tumour or how much of the bowel would need to be removed. He wanted to do the surgery in the morning because he liked to do the 'big jobs' in the morning. Small comfort. But I had to get the problem removed to repair my body. It didn't occur to me that I may die. I accepted that whatever the outcome, it would be right for me.

The Operation

The surgery was two weeks later. The first procedure on entering hospital was x-ray, then came blood tests. At 3 p.m. the day before the operation a nurse brought in the Glycoprep. Yuk! She commiserated with me about having to take the muck, but that was no help to me. She was not the one who had to swallow the stuff, I was!

On the morning of the operation the anaesthetist gave me one of those fetching gowns to put on, checked my hands for a suitable vein, then put a needle into that vein. I thought I was being particularly brave! I was given the pre-med injection through this needle instead of an injection in my backside. What a relief.

I have been told that the operation took 4 and 1/2 hours. I don't know how much longer than that I was out. When I was fully conscious the surgeon came to see me. He told me the surgery had been successful, that the cancer had been encapsulated and they had been able to remove the whole thing. It had not penetrated the bowel wall so I would not need chemo-therapy or any further treatment. I was fortunate. I had a sense of relief and release, but I had not considered any other result. It was a process I had to experience for some reason or higher purpose.

During the operation they had attached a colostomy bag and a tube through a small hole in my side attached to a bag which seemed to have vacuum pressure to drain the wound. The colostomy meant I didn't have to ask for a pan or go to the toilet. I was on a drip and my body was functioning normally so there was waste to be removed.

When the drip was removed ten days after the operation I was given a medicine glass with 2 mls of water to drink every two hours while they checked my bowel function. The amount of water was gradually increased when it became obvious that my bowel was healing well. After this my diet varied a little - jelly and soup were added. Although I was not interested in food I realised I had to eat.

Once at home my appetite was poor for about a month. Tomato soup and toast were a major part of my diet for that time. To get back to eating normally took months. There are foods I cannot eat now that I used to enjoy, fatty things mostly make me feel ill.

Following the operation I had regular blood tests and check ups with the surgeon. Cancer cells show up in blood as an early warning. All the tests have been clear. I had the final check five years to the day from the surgery, but I have colonoscopies every three years as a preventive measure.

Recovery

I went to a GP/Natural Therapist who suggested I increase my dosage of Vitamin C to help my body recover from the effects of surgery and anaesthetics, and to take Selenium. I also added a small handful of almonds plus a megadophilus supplement to my diet to help my intestines to recover. I am eating more fish and take Omega 3 and Omega 6 oils, together with Vitamin B, especially B12. I have noticed a further benefit from these - less susceptibility to colds and flu and less stress.

Bowel cancer does not strike only the elderly or those who have a family history of it. It can strike anyone at any age. I have a friend whose 17 year old daughter contracted it. A major point to be recognised is that it may appear at any time in any person. It does not attack either sex in preference to the other, nor does it develop after a particular age, although I have been told that it is more prevalent in older people.

The way to recover from bowel cancer, to catch it in time to conquer it, is to take notice of every symptom. If, as happened to me, you pass a blood clot, have yourself checked. If, as happened to an older lady I know, you feel constipated all the time, or your bowel movements spurt, have yourself checked.

It is better to be safe than sorry. Your local GP can give a preliminary examination. I know it may seem embarrassing or uncomfortable to some people to discuss this area of your body and your bodily functions but it is worth it. It really is worth it.

Talking to various people about my experience of the cancer and how it has affected my life, I am uncovering feelings of my early years. I have been told that the person developing cancer has been bottling up emotional pain over many years, that a dis-ease within you causes a disease of the body. A bad diet including a lot of refined foods, sugars and processed flours, may be a trigger for some illnesses. However, I don't think anyone has yet successfully explained how one gets cancer.

It is only now, five years down the track, I realise I went through rather a lot, both emotionally and physically, following the diagnosis. I have had to adjust to the physical problems caused by the bowel cancer, and to come to terms with my body being so damaged by the surgery to remove it. I had imagined the wound to be a long straight line. However, I did not realise just how long or how wide it was until I summoned up enough courage to look at it. It was as if not looking at it meant it didn't happen, that the surgeon had been able to operate so as not to damage the surface of the skin. I didn't take this idea much further. I carefully avoided looking at my stomach area.

There was a feeling of grief on first seeing the wound. It was a shock to see the damage to my body. The colour of the scar has eased from angry dark red to a paler dark pink over the five years, but it and the staple marks are with me for the rest of my life. My scar is a reminder to me that we cannot take life for granted. I still look at it with amazement. It did happen to me. I went through a major operation for the removal of a cancerous growth. I would not have survived but for seeing that blood clot and doing something about it.

Thoughts that I may not have time 'later' to do the things that I had been putting off only came to me as I heard of people who had died from not having discovered their cancer early enough, or not taking note of the symptoms they were experiencing.

My feelings at discovering that I had bowel cancer and that I would have to be operated on were of total disbelief. For most of my life, anything negative that has happened to me, I suppressed. The cancer would not be suppressed - it wanted to be looked at. My belief now is that I went through the experience of having and recovering successfully from bowel cancer so that I am able to write about it from a positive viewpoint to help others.

Candida

The fungus known, as Candida Albicans is a yeast-like organism, which is a common inhabitant of the mouth, throat, intestines and vagina. Normally the healthy bacteria of the gut, compete with the candida and keep it under control, so that it exists happily without causing any health problems.

Candida can become a problem in the gut and other mucous membranes of the body if the diet is incorrect, inflammation exists, or after the use of antibiotic drugs, steroids and the oral contraceptive pill. As the candida yeast flourishes the bowels become an overactive fermentation tank. This causes excessive gas, abdominal bloating and irregular bowel actions. There may be a thick white vaginal discharge and the tongue may develop a white coating associated with white patches in the mouth.

The yeast Candida albicans can change its form from a simple non-invasive cell to an invasive mycelial form with tendrils (tentacles) *see diagram below*.

These tendrils grow like roots and can penetrate the wall of the bowel, and act like a leaking pipe through which waste products and toxins can enter into the bloodstream, bypassing the liver. The liver is unable to get to these toxins which can then cause symptoms such as fatigue, allergies and mysterious ill health.

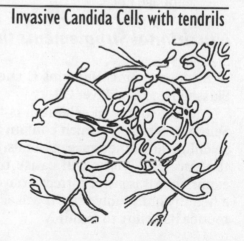

Invasive Candida Cells with tendrils

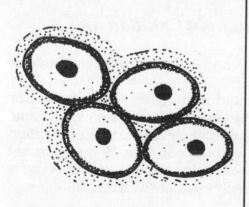

Non-invasive Candida Cells

Anti-Candida Diet

• **Avoid** bread that is not yeast free, yeast extracts such as vegemite and marmite, dairy products, vinegar, alcohol, pickles and preserves, jams, canned fruits and vegetables, dried fruits, peanuts, melons, any fruit that is mouldy (best to remove skin on all fruits if you have candida), all foods containing white sugar and flour, lollies, cakes and biscuits, sweet drinks, and any foods containing malt as an additive.

• **Raw sugar** is a problem for those with candida. It may be possible to use a good quality honey because honey contains natural antibiotics that stop fungi from growing. Some people with severe candida might need to avoid honey and all other sweeteners.

• **Fruit** can be eaten provided it is very fresh and free of mouldy areas. Restrict the intake of fruits to no more than 2 to 3 pieces daily if you find that you are unable to control candida. In those with severe candida, fruit should be avoided for the first three months.

• **Oat, rice or soy milk** may be used, however, be sure to avoid brands that contain malt, or maltodextrin.

• **The diet should be high in fibre** and raw vegetables to make sure that the contents of the bowel are emptied regularly. This prevents candida from building up in the bowel and causing fermentation.

• **Soy yoghurt contains friendly lactobacillus bacteria**, which help to fight candida and can be consumed regularly, however avoid those brands that contain sugar or fruit. You can also take powders containing lactobacillus and these must be kept refrigerated.

• **Foods that have natural antibiotic properties** will fight candida very effectively if they are eaten regularly. The best ones are raw garlic (finely chopped, grated or juiced), onions, leeks, and radishes, cruciferous vegetables (broccoli, Brussels sprouts, cauliflower, cabbage), fresh gingerroot (finely chopped or grated) and raw cabbage juice.

Nutritional Supplements that fight Candida are:

Selenium, Zinc, Vitamins C and A and essential fatty acids such as Flaxseed and Cod Liver Oil.

A good source of selenium is found in designer yeast powders or Selemite B tablets, which contain Brewer's yeast, fortified with organic selenium and other trace minerals. Some people have the misconception that Brewer's yeast will cause or worsen candida, however in my experience this is not correct. I have found that because Brewer's yeast is a healthy or friendly yeast it will actually compete with the candida and reduce its ability to multiply.

Herbs that will help to Fight Candida are:

Golden Seal, Aloe Vera and best of all Olive Leaf extract, which is available in capsule form.

Medical treatment for candida may require the use of high dose mycostatin tablets and/or intravenous, high dose vitamin C.

High Cholesterol

The subject of high cholesterol is rather controversial and often poorly understood by those who have it. Cholesterol is a natural substance that is vital to life, being found in the brain, nerves, liver, bile and indeed in most cells of the body. Without cholesterol the glands could not produce steroid hormones such as cortisone and sex hormones, as cholesterol is converted into steroid hormones. Another thing that may surprise you, is that the liver makes 80% of the total body cholesterol, and only 20% comes from dietary sources. Disturbed liver function can cause serious problems with the regulation of total body cholesterol levels.

Cholesterol needs to be transported from the liver around the body in the bloodstream to get to the cells that require it. It cannot travel by itself and must be carried by specialised proteins called lipoproteins. You have probably heard of these lipoproteins by the names of low-density lipoproteins (LDLs), and high-density lipoproteins (HDLs). LDLs are sometimes called "bad cholesterol," and HDLs are known as "good cholesterol". These reputations are derived from the fact that LDLs are heavily laden with cholesterol while they are transporting it from the liver to all the body cells. HDLs carry much less cholesterol and their main function is to scavenge excess unwanted cholesterol from the cells and the bloodstream and carry it back to the liver. If the liver is working efficiently everything remains in proper balance and blood cholesterol levels are easily controlled. If the liver does not manufacture sufficient HDLs, blood cholesterol levels will rise which can form fatty plaque, lining the blood vessel walls. This is the origin of cardiovascular diseases such as heart attacks, some forms of high blood pressure and strokes.

Some people become very alarmed if they discover that their total cholesterol levels are high, however this may not be dangerous depending upon whether the total cholesterol is made up of mainly the good HDLs or the bad LDLs. The respective amounts of these things can be accurately measured in a sample of blood taken after you have fasted for 12 hours. Only fasting specimens of blood will give accurate and meaningful levels of cholesterol.

If your total cholesterol level is elevated, **see table on page 148**, it is far more serious if your HDLs are abnormally low or borderline, and the bulk of your excess cholesterol consists of the bad LDLs. Make sure you ask your doctor to look into your balance of LDL and HDL cholesterol.

Normal ranges of the different types of cholesterol as determined by blood tests

Units of Measurement	Australian mmol/L	American mg/dl
Total Cholesterol	3.9-5.5	up to 200
HDL Cholesterol -male - female	0.8-1.7 0.9-2.1	45-50 50-60
LDL Cholesterol	1.7-4.5	below 126

There is no longer any doubt that an abnormally high cholesterol level (mainly LDL cholesterol), is a major risk factor for heart disease, the number one killer of adults in the West. Lowering cholesterol and in particular LDL levels, reduces this risk. A major study on cholesterol levels and coronary artery disease conducted by the National Heart, Lung and Blood Institute of America, found that a 1% reduction in cholesterol level leads to a 2% reduction in coronary heart disease and its fatal consequences.

Ideally your total cholesterol levels should be around the middle or lower end of the normal ranges in the table above, however if they are towards the upper end of the normal range there is no concern if the HDL cholesterol levels are plentiful. HDL cholesterol is protective against heart disease and is also important in the healthy function of the brain. Indeed approximately two thirds of the brain's weight consists of HDL cholesterol. HDL also exists in the walls of arteries and acts to lubricate the arterial wall to facilitate the easy flow of blood. This helps to keep blood pressure under control. So if you have high levels of HDL cholesterol you are fortunate (even if they are over 60 mg/dl or 2.1 mmol/L), because this is heart protective. Low levels of HDL cholesterol (see table above) are dangerous, even if your total cholesterol is normal. It is interesting to know that very low total cholesterol levels are not always desirable either and you do not need to aim for the lowest possible level. Very low levels of cholesterol may be associated with higher risks of stroke, cancer and depression. It is more important to aim for the right balance of the good HDLs to the bad LDLs. The liver filter and the liver's metabolic pathways control this balance, which is why it is so important to have a healthy efficient liver. As we say "love your liver, and live longer!"

What should you do if you have abnormally high levels of cholesterol or low HDL cholesterol?

- **Follow** the vital principles of the Liver Cleansing Diet
- **Take** a good liver tonic regularly *see page 28*
- **Eat** plenty of high fibre foods (wholegrains, cereals, seeds, legumes, bran, raw foods) Aim for 50-60 grams (1.8 - 2oz) of dietary fibre daily *see page124*
- **Exercise** is vital, especially of the aerobic variety which will raise HDLs and lower total cholesterol.
- **Use** specific anti-fat foods and condiments from your kitchen, which fight cholesterol. These are chilli, capsicums, garlic, onions, leeks, radishes, fenugreek, fresh gingerroot, tumeric, lecithin granules and Brewer's yeast.
- **Take** Chromium picolinate 200mcg daily.
- **Drink** plenty of water - 2 to 3 litres daily and drink one glass of mixed raw vegetable juice daily.
- **Take** Vitamin C 2000 mg daily.

Other specific supplements that you may find very effective for stubbornly high cholesterol can be tried. These should be taken under the supervision of your health care provider.

These are:

Pantethine 600 to 1200 mg daily (eg 300mg three times daily with food). Some studies have found this to be helpful and it is free of side effects.
Nicotinic acid (preferably in the long acting form) must only be tried under medical supervision, as although it can be very effective it may cause unpleasant side effects if excess doses are used. Start with 250mg daily with meals and gradually build up to 500mg three times daily with meals.
Acetyl-L-carnitine 500 mg daily on an empty stomach or L-**Carnitine plus L-cysteine plus L-methionine**, 500mg of each daily on an empty stomach.

There are a number of cholesterol-lowering drugs commonly prescribed by doctors, which can be expensive and have unpleasant and even serious side effects. Make sure you ask your doctor about possible side effects, and even better check the side effect list that comes with the product information. This will help you to understand why nutritional medicine is so much safer and in most cases more effective in the long term. I believe that you should try natural therapies, dietary and life-style changes before taking these drugs, but of course it's up to you!

Remember to take care of your liver, avoid animal fats and fried foods, and eat raw salads and fibre, and cholesterol levels will gradually and naturally come down and balance out.

There is a small group of people who have inherited a metabolic defect in cholesterol metabolism, and these cases are called Familial Hypercholesterolaemia. These people often have extremely high and dangerous levels of cholesterol, which cannot be controlled with diet alone and will require long-term drug therapy.

Pancreatitis

The term pancreatitis refers to inflammation of the pancreas gland, which is situated deeply in the upper abdominal area. It may be acute, severe and life threatening, or chronic and intermittent. It usually produces pain in the upper abdomen, which often spreads deeper into the back between the shoulder blades. The pain can vary from mild and grumbling, to sudden and excruciating, and is usually accompanied by nausea and vomiting.

The possible causes of pancreatitis are gallstones, alcohol abuse, viral infections, poor blood supply, some drug side effects, and sometimes are unknown. If the cause of an illness is unknown, it is called "idiopathic". In most cases of idiopathic pancreatitis, there will be problems with the function of the liver and gallbladder, and in particular the bile may contain excessive sludge and toxic waste products which inflame the pancreatic duct. The pancreas can also become inflamed from being overworked in those who ingest too much rich food high in animal fats and proteins and refined sugars. This forces the pancreas to produce excessive amounts of digestive enzymes, and if the ducts within the pancreas are swollen or compressed with fat, these digestive enzymes can become trapped inside the pancreas and start to digest the pancreas itself. This process, known as auto-digestion of the pancreas, causes great pain, and damages the cells of the pancreas. This may result in cysts developing inside the pancreas.

If you have pancreatitis I recommend the following:
- Small frequent meals are better than large meals.
- Follow the principles of the Liver Cleansing Diet.
- Avoid alcohol, fatty foods, fried foods and refined sugars.
- Avoid unnecessary drugs and painkillers.
- Digestive enzymes-pancreatin - 2-4 grams with each meal will reduce the work load of the pancreas.
- Magnesium Complete - 1 tablet with every meal.
- Vitamin C - 500 mg with every meal.
- Vitamin E - 500 i.u. with every meal.
- A good liver tonic in powder form, one teaspoon stirred into juice twice daily before food.

Diabetes Mellitus

Diabetes is a common problem in Western affluent societies where people consume excess amounts of refined sugars, carbohydrates and fats. Indeed because of incorrect diet and lifestyle, the incidence of diabetes is increasing and has approximately tripled since 1953.

There are two types of diabetes:

Type 1 - this type is more common in children and young adults and accounts for around 5% of all cases of diabetes.

In Type 1 diabetes, the pancreas gland stops producing the hormone insulin, which is needed to control the body's utilisation of sugar (glucose). This may be genetic, autoimmune or caused by viruses or toxins that attack and damage the pancreas. The treatment of Type 1 diabetes requires the administration of daily injections of the hormone insulin, which will control blood sugar levels.

Type II - this type is far more common and represents 95% of all diabetics. Type II diabetics are often overweight and can have great difficulty losing weight.

The incidence of fatty liver is higher in those with Type II diabetes. Liver dysfunction is common which can cause unstable blood sugar levels. When the blood sugar drops too low, very strong cravings for sugar make it difficult to stick to a low sugar diet. A healthy liver manufactures a substance called glucose tolerance factor (GTF) from glutathione and chromium. GTF helps the hormone insulin to regulate blood sugar levels efficiently. Left over sugars are stored in the liver in the form of glycogen, which acts as a storage depot for sugar that can be released quickly into the blood stream when you need it. I have long been aware of the significance of unhealthy liver function in the genesis of Type II diabetes, and yet this is an association that receives insufficient research. As I have said before, the liver is still the "forgotten organ" in many common disease states. This will change over the next decade, if not sooner.

It is very important to improve liver function in this type of diabetes by following the principles of the Liver Cleansing Diet, and taking a good liver tonic.

In Type II diabetes the pancreas retains its ability to secrete insulin and indeed in many cases there is an overproduction of insulin. This does not really help with the control of blood sugar because there is a resistance to the effect of the insulin, and blood sugar levels remain high. These people have often overworked their pancreas by unwittingly consuming excess amounts of refined sugars and damaged fats. In response the pancreas pumps out huge amounts of insulin which does not control the metabolic imbalance. It is almost as if the body gets accustomed to the very high insulin levels becoming resistant or insensitive to them. These high levels of insulin can increase appetite, which contributes to the high incidence of obesity in Type II diabetics.

Type II diabetes can present with vague symptoms such as fatigue, aches and pains, excess thirst, blurred vision, poor concentration and memory, loss of hair on the legs, and fatty lumps under the skin. Analysis of the urine with a simple dipstick in the doctor's rooms or pharmacy, can often detect unsuspected diabetes.

Type II diabetes can be effectively treated with correct diet and exercise, and if necessary, weight loss. The dietary and medical treatment of diabetes is somewhat controversial and there are differing opinions. For example some dieticians allow diabetics to use artificial sweeteners (eg aspartame) and hydrogenated vegetable oils (eg margarine). I do not agree with this at all and these things will not help your liver or pancreas to recover. I would avoid these things and use natural foods containing healing nutrients instead.

One researcher Mark Sorensen, believes that excessive dietary cholesterol causes diabetes, and he recommends a diet high in complex carbohydrates and low in cholesterol and refined sugars. Another well known American medical doctor and author by the name of Dr. Robert Atkins, recommends a diet high in protein (including animal protein), low in complex carbohydrates, and devoid of any refined sugar and carbohydrate. Both of these doctors have achieved good results in their patients. They both used a moderate exercise program, nutritional supplements and low calorie diets.

I have found that over 80% of my diabetic patients achieved excellent results after reducing their body weight and keeping on with regular exercise. I did find that it was much easier for them to lose weight if they first improved their liver function.

Before I give you my dietary recommendations for diabetes I would like to explain something about carbohydrates. Carbohydrates supply the body with energy and are found mainly in plant foods such as legumes (beans, lentils and peas), seeds, nuts, grains, fruits and vegetables. Milk and its products are the only animal foods that contain significant amounts of carbohydrates.

Dietary carbohydrates are the major source of the body's glucose, which fuels every cell.

Carbohydrates can be divided into 3 groups:

Simple carbohydrates: or simple sugars which include fructose (sugar found in all fruit), sucrose (table sugar) and lactose (milk sugar), are the most common. In their natural state they coexist with vitamins and minerals, which helps the body to use them efficiently. Simple carbohydrates are converted into glucose, which is the body's fuel.

Complex carbohydrates: these are also made up of sugars, however the molecules are attached together to form longer, more complex structures. Complex carbohydrates are part of starches and fibre. Good sources of complex carbohydrates are legumes, cereals, whole grains, seeds, raw nuts and vegetables. Complex carbohydrates are converted into glucose and are combined with vitamins and minerals, which enables the body to use them efficiently.

Refined carbohydrates: these are found in processed foods such as white sugar and white flour. Foods high in refined carbohydrates are lollies, candies, sweet biscuits and cakes (made with white flour and sugar), white bread, pastas made with white flour, fizzy sweet soft drinks and some processed foods. They are converted to glucose, but because they are devoid of vitamins and minerals, the body finds them difficult to metabolise. They make your liver and pancreas work too hard, which in the long term will stress these organs and may lead to disease. They are more likely to cause unstable blood sugar levels, obesity and diabetes.

My dietary recommendations for diabetics are:

• Follow a high fibre diet. Foods high in fibre are shown on *page 124*. Especially good high fibre foods for diabetics are legumes (beans, peas, lentils), whole oats, buckwheat, apples and all varieties of green vegetables.

• Eat plenty of raw vegetables, as this will improve liver function and aid weight loss. We have many yummy salad recipes in this book which can be used with our nice salad dressings, *see page 190*.

• Use complex carbohydrates (see above) instead of simple or refined carbohydrates. This will stabilise blood sugar levels and aid weight loss. Generally it is recommended that 60% of your total daily calories come from complex carbohydrates.

• Avoid refined carbohydrates as much as possible (see above)

• Ensure that you eat foods containing essential fatty acids, such as oily fish, avocados, flaxseed, other seeds and raw nuts, lecithin and cold pressed vegetable oils. Eggs are a good source of lecithin and protein and can be eaten in moderation by diabetics. Essential fatty acids help to reduce blood clots and cardiovascular complications of diabetes. Essential fatty acids are vitally important for diabetics, as they will reduce the risk of diabetic neuropathy, which can affect the limbs and the eyes.

• Drink plenty of water and if desired herbal teas and herbal coffee such as dandelion, nettle and ginger.

• Avoid a high intake of animal fats such as fatty meats, high fat dairy products, fried foods and animal skins and offal. Try to get free-range chicken for its lower fat content. Avoid all dairy products. Generally speaking fats should not exceed 30% of the total calorie intake and it is important to try and follow this. However, I believe the type of fat you are eating is more important than the quantity. It is not necessary to follow a very low fat diet (ie less than 20% of calorie intake) because this may lead to fatigue and hunger and has not

been shown to improve the outcome of diabetes.
• Avoid alcohol except for the occasional moderate use of good quality aged red wine.

Helpful Supplements for Diabetics

• **Vitamin E** - 1000 i.u. daily to reduce vascular complications.
• **Vitamin C** - 1000 mg two to three times daily to reduce vascular problems.
• **Trace minerals** such as chromium, selenium, zinc, manganese and magnesium. Selenium yeast powders are a form of high mineral Brewer's yeast and can be helpful for diabetics. Brewer's yeast is high in B group vitamins, which help to stabilise blood sugar levels. Some of these powders contain the naturally sweet herb Stevia that is safe to use in small amounts.
• **Chromium picolinate** - in a relatively high daily dose of 400 to 600 mcg has been shown to improve the effect of insulin in a significant percentage of diabetics.
• **L-carnitine** - 500 mg twice daily, on an empty stomach to help energy production in cells.
• **Coenzyme Q 10** - 50 - 100 mg daily to aid cellular energy production
• **Magnesium Complete** - 3 tablets daily
• **Manganese** - 5 mg daily
• **Zinc** - 30 to 50 mg daily
• **B complex** - one tablet daily helps glucose metabolism and peripheral nerves.
• **The herbs** Bilberry and Ginkgo biloba contain bioflavonoids that aid the peripheral circulation. They can be taken in 8-week courses from time to time and you may find that your vision improves.
• **Raw garlic** is superb for diabetics aiding both the liver and pancreas, and helping to prevent the vascular complications of diabeties. The best way to use raw garlic is to chop or grate it finely, or squeeze juice out in a garlic press. Mix with your salad and cooked vegetables and meat. For the socially paranoid, odourless garlic capsules can be used, however although they are worthwhile they are not as effective as raw garlic.
• **Lipoic acid** , also known as alpha lipoic acid has been demonstrated to be an effective compound for improving glucose utilisation and reducing the glycosylation of proteins. It is excellent for diabetics and those with impaired glucose tolerance or insulin resistance. Dosage required may vary from 100mg to 1000mg daily. Ref. 22

In long standing diabetes the pancreas may be "worn out" and unable to produce sufficient digestive enzymes. Taking a supplement of pancreatic enzymes such as pancreatin, will help digestion and absorption of vital nutrients.

Food Allergies

Some people have multiple food and chemical sensitivities, which makes it difficult for them to follow a set diet. These problems are always associated with reduced ability of the liver to breakdown chemicals and proteins (antigens) in the detoxification pathways. Therefore it is always necessary to improve liver function in such cases, and the use of a powerful natural liver tonic as discussed on *page 28* will improve the detoxification pathways in the liver. This will gradually reduce the unpleasant reactions to foods and chemicals suffered by these patients.

As well as a liver tonic, it is useful to take extra amounts of the amino acid Taurine and Vitamin C, to improve the phase two-detoxification pathway in the liver. Doses required are Taurine 1000mg three times daily with meals, and Vitamin C 1000mg three times daily with meals.

These patients must source a reliable supplier of organically produced meats, fruits and vegetables (*see page 287)* and use a high quality water purifier as their overloaded liver cannot cope with environmental toxins. They need to consume foods that are high in natural sulphur compounds to support the liver's detoxification pathways. The best foods for this purpose are garlic, onions, leeks, radishes, cruciferous vegetables (broccoli, cabbage, Brussels sprouts and cauliflower) and eggs. If they are allergic to any of these foods they should be replaced with other foods high in sulphur to which they are not allergic.

The adrenal glands also need to be supported in cases of severe chemical and food sensitivity, as they may not be producing sufficient steroid hormones such as cortisone, pregnenolone and DHEA (dehydroepiandrosterone), and this will increase the severity of allergic reactions. Thankfully it is easy to test the levels of these adrenal hormones with a blood test, and also to replace these natural hormones in the form of lozenges or creams. For more details on the treatment of adrenal problems with natural hormones, you can refer to my book titled "Boost Your Energy". The adrenal glands can also be helped with supplemental amounts of essential fatty acids (good sources are cod liver oil and flaxseed oil) and vitamin E 1000 i.u. daily. Vitamin B 5, also known as pantothenic acid, can strengthen the adrenal glands, and the dose required is 100 mg three times daily.

Food allergies are also often triggered when only partially digested foods are absorbed from the intestines, which may occur in those with an inflamed lining of the small and large intestine. This is also known as "leaky gut syndrome." The liver finds it much harder to breakdown large molecules in only partially digested foods and this will overload the liver and can cause food intolerances. In this situation it is vital to take some form of digestive enzymes in the middle of eating your meal. Pancreatic enzymes are available in tablet and powder form, and contain the full complement of digestive enzymes to break down food particles into small easily absorbed molecules. You may need to adjust the dosage under the supervision of your practitioner as some people require much higher doses than others.

It is essential that patients with severe food and chemical intolerances consult a specialist in allergies who will perform extensive tests to accurately determine the things that must be avoided. The most common foods to cause allergies are dairy products, gluten (found in wheat, rye, barley and oats), salicylates (found in most plants and herbs - *see page 160*) and shellfish. Artificial sweeteners and food additives, can build up in the body, eventually causing severe allergic reactions. The most common offenders are MSG (monosodium glutamate), aspartame, sulphites, benzoates and nitrites, and artificial colourings. Check labels to see if these things are present and if so, avoid them.

Laboratory tests can be done through your doctor to check for food allergies. The most reliable test uses a blood sample to measure antibody proteins (IgG) that your body may be making against foods to which you are allergic. It is possible to test your reaction to many different foods using this IgG food panel test.

Those with severe manifestations of allergies such as asthma, severe swelling of the lips and throat, hives, and those on cortisone, can suffer fatal reactions to chemicals, foods and insect bites. These people should remain under the supervision of an allergist, and carry a syringe of adrenalin for self-injection should an anaphylactic reaction occur and immediate help is unavailable.

If you want to follow the Liver Cleansing Diet recipes and yet feel apprehensive because you have multiple food allergies, I suggest that you check each recipe carefully before trying it. If there are foods in some of the recipes to which you are allergic, it is easy for you to substitute the offending ingredient with another ingredient to which you are not allergic.

Substitute Foods for Food Allergies

ALLERGY	SUBSTITUTES
Cows Milk	Soy, Rice, Almond, Coconut and Oat Milk
Butter	Tahini, Houmus, Pesto (cheese free) Nut Spreads, Honey, Garlic Paste, Tomato Paste, Miso, Avocado, Olive paste
Cheese	Soy Cheese - grill or grate, Avocado
Yoghurt	Soy Yoghurt
Ice Cream, Cream	Fruit Sorbet, Fruit Iceblocks, Tofu Ice-cream
Chocolate	Carob, Halva
Wheat	Rice, Corn, Quinoa, Buckwheat, Teff Flours and pastas made from Soy, Millet, flaxseed, Cornmeal, Amaranth, Lentils

Self Test For Food Allergies

This involves measuring your pulse rate after eating the suspected food. **Measure** your pulse rate at your wrist while you are sitting in a relaxed state before eating. Normally the pulse rate will be between 55 to 75 beats per minute at this time.

Then consume the food that you think you may be allergic to and stay seated and relaxed. After 20 minutes measure your pulse rate again at the wrist. If your pulse rate has increased by more than 10 beats per minute (ie. gone from 60 to 72 beats per minute), you are probably intolerant to this food. This is all the more likely if you feel unwell, dizzy or nauseated as your pulse rate increases. **Omit** this food from your diet for 8 weeks and see if your health improves. You can then retest yourself with this food again and see if the adverse reaction persists. If it persists then permanently omit this food from your diet.

Tests For Bowel and Digestive Function

If you believe that you may have a digestive or bowel problem it is a good idea to see a specialist in gastrointestinal disorders, known as a gastroenterologist. These doctors will take an extensive history of your eating patterns, symptoms and bowel actions. The most serious problems to exclude are malignant tumours of the stomach and bowels, which become far more common as we age. This is why it is important to have thorough investigations early on if you develop any change in bowel actions, unexplained weight loss or abdominal pains.

Specialised tests known as a **"Complete Diagnostic Stool Analysis"** (CDSA) can be done by **Analytical Reference Laboratories** in Melbourne, Australia, and your health care provider can arrange these tests for you. Their phone number is **(613) 9328 3586**. In the USA these tests can be done at the **Great Smokies Laboratories**, Phone: **(828) 285 223.**

The CDSA is divided into panel A and panel B.

Panel A assesses the overall appearance of your bowel actions (stools), as well as checking them for blood cells and fat globules. It also measures the stools for markers of food digestion and absorption, such as triglyceride fats, chymotrypsin enzyme, meat fibres, vegetable cells and fibres, acid-base balance, and short chain fatty acids such as valerate and iso-butyrate, long chain fatty acids, cholesterol and total faecal fat. Panel A will give your doctor a very good evaluation of your ability to digest and absorb a wide range of food groups. This is important because even though you may have an excellent diet, you may not be able to extract the vital nutrients from it if your liver, pancreas, stomach or intestines are malfunctioning.

Panel B assesses the population of microorganisms in your gut. This is done using microscopy and cultures to look for parasites, bacteria and fungi that may be unwelcome inhabitants of your stomach and intestines. These intruders may be robbing you of vital nutrients and causing inflammation of your bowels, which is rather rude seeing they don't pay any rent!

It is also possible to test for common stomach bacteria called Helicobacter pylori, which are a cause of gastric and duodenal ulcers. Testing for the Helicobacter Direct Antigen in the stools can do this.

Colonoscopy

This involves passing through the anus a thin flexible tube that visualises the lining of the entire colon and rectum, and transmits the picture to a television screen. Samples (biopsies) can be taken from suspicious looking areas of the bowel to enable accurate diagnosis. It is done under mild intravenous sedation and takes around 30 minutes. The test is usually not uncomfortable. The colon needs to be cleansed with laxatives beforehand to enable an accurate assessment. Colonoscopy is the most accurate way to diagnose the cause of bowel symptoms and to screen for cancer and bowel polyps. Bowel polyps can be removed via this procedure. There is a slight risk of perforation of the colon (1 in 2000 cases) during colonoscopy.

Sigmoidoscopy

This is similar to colonoscopy, however the flexible tube that is passed up into the bowel is much shorter and can only assess the lower part of the large bowel (rectum and sigmoid colon). It is usually done in your doctor's office and does not usually require intravenous sedation. This test takes around 5 minutes and may cause a feeling of gas and slight cramping. An enema is required to cleanse the bowel beforehand.

Barium Enema X ray

This is an X-ray examination of the large bowel (colon and rectum) which enables the doctor to assess the shape, size and smoothness of the outline of your large bowel. The X-ray is performed after you receive an enema to insert barium (a chalky radio-opaque) liquid into the rectum which will contrast and outline the wall of the large bowel. A barium enema will show up enlargement of the large bowel and irregularities of the bowel wall and bowel pockets known as diverticula. It can also reveal muscular spasm (spastic colon) in the wall of the large bowel.

In some cases of severe constipation a barium enema X ray will reveal a huge dilated colon with extra loops of unwanted bowel (redundant bowel), and this is known as a "megacolon". A barium enema may show some types of bowel cancer, however it can also miss small cancers, and for this reason a colonoscopy is a far more accurate way to exclude bowel cancer. Sometimes a barium swallow is done to outline the stomach and small intestines.

Salicylate Intolerance

Salicylates are "aspirin-like substances" that exist naturally in plants and herbs. In some people with liver dysfunction, an intolerance to salicylates gradually develops because the liver is unable to break down dietary salicylates. Salicylate intolerance can cause many symptoms such as hives, hay fever, asthma, skin rashes, headaches and irritable bowel syndrome. If you suspect that you have a salicylate intolerance consult an allergy specialist to confirm this. Salicylate intolerance can gradually be overcome by improving liver function through correct diet and taking supplemental taurine. It is also necessary to take a liver tonic that can improve the phase one and two detoxification pathways in the liver. This will help to break down salicylates.

If you are allergic to salicylates the table on *pages 161 to 162,* will help you to choose low salicylate food alternatives, which can be substituted in the recipes. You can flavour and season the recipes with the herbs that are low in salicylates. You will note from the table that garlic is low in salicylates. Garlic is a very good food to eat for those wanting to overcome a salicylate allergy/intolerance. This is because garlic helps the phase two-detoxification pathway in the liver, which helps the liver to breakdown salicylates.

You may be aware that many older persons with vascular problems take low dose aspirin tablets to thin the blood. Aspirin is synthetic salicylate. All salicylates thin the blood by reducing platelet stickiness, which reduces the tendency to form blood clots.

By eating foods high in salicylates, such as cayenne, curry, paprika, tumeric, cummin, mustard, ginger, tomatoes, radish, olives, capsicum and hot peppers (chillis) it is also possible to keep the blood thinner, thereby reducing the tendency to form unwanted blood clots. This is good for people with cardiovascular disease. See the table for a full list of foods high and very high in salicylates to give you more variety. For people who do not have salicylate intolerance, foods high in salicylates are extremely beneficial for the health of the cardiovascular system.

Food Salicylate Content Table

Fruits

NEGLIGIBLE	LOW	MODERATE	HIGH	VERY HIGH
Pear (peeled)	Pawpaw Golden & delicious apple	Pear (with peel) Loquat Custard apple Red Delicious apple Persimmon Lemon Fig Rhubarb Mango Tamarillo	Passionfruit Mulberry Tangello Grapefruit Avocado Peach Mandarin Granny Smith apple Nectarine Watermelon Lychee Jonathan apple	Sultana (dried) Prune Raisin (dried) Raspberry Redcurrant Loganberry Blackcurrant Youngberry Date Cherry Blueberry Orange Kiwi fruit Boysenberry Guava Blackberry Cranberry Apricot Strawberry Rockmelon Grape Plum Pineapple

Vegetables

NEGLIGIBLE	LOW	MODERATE	HIGH	VERY HIGH
Potato (peeled) Lettuce Celery Cabbage Bamboo shoot Swede Dried beans Dried peas Red Lentils Brown Lentils	Green bean Redcabbage Brussels sprouts Mung bean sprouts Green pea Leek Shallot Chive Choko	Broccoli Sweet potato Parsnip Mushroom Carrot Beetroot Marrow Spinach Onion Cauliflower Turnip Asparagus Sweetcorn Pumpkin	Eggplant Watercress Cucumber Broad bean Alfalfa sprouts	Tomato products Gherkin Endive Champignon Radish Olive Capsicum Zucchini Chicory Hot pepper

Nuts

NEGLIGIBLE	LOW	MODERATE	HIGH	VERY HIGH
Poppyseed	Cashews	Pistachio Pinenut Macadamia Walnut Brazil		Almond Water chestnut

Nuts cont.

NEGLIGIBLE	LOW	MODERATE	HIGH	VERY HIGH
		Coconut Peanut Hazelnut Pecan Sunflower seeds Sesame		

Sweets

NEGLIGIBLE	LOW	MODERATE	HIGH	VERY HIGH
White sugar Maple syrup Cocoa Carob	Golden syrup Caramels	Molasses		Licquorice Peppermints Honey

Herbs and Spices

NEGLIGIBLE	LOW	MODERATE	HIGH	VERY HIGH
	Vanilla Garlic Parsley Saffron Malt vinegar Soy sauce Tandori		Cinnamon Cardamom Black pepper Pimiento Ginger Allspice Clove Nutmeg Caraway White vinegar Bay Leaf Whitepepper	Cayenne Aniseed Sage Mace Curry Paprika Thyme Dill Tumeric Worcestershire sauce Vegemite Marmite Rosemary Oregano Garam masala Mixed herbs Cumin Canella Tarragon Mustard Five spice Mint

Alcohol

NEGLIGIBLE	LOW	MODERATE	HIGH	VERY HIGH
Gin Whiskey Vodka		Cider Beer Sherry Brandy		Liqueur Port Wine Rum

Section Three - The Recipes

Housekeeping with Audrey Tea ...164

Beverages ...168
       Juices, Smoothies and Teas

Breakfasts ...174

Soups ...181

Dips, Spreads and Dressings ...190

Salads, Sides and Snacks ...193

Vegetable Mains ...212

Poultry ...230

Seafood ...242

Meat ...258

Sweets, Treats and Cakes ...263

Appendix Section Three
       Conversion Chart ...285
       Organic Food Suppliers ...287
       Contact Details ...291
       Glossary ...295

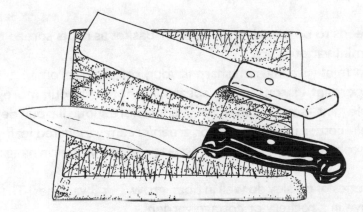

a herb garden

A herb garden can provide you with fresh herbs and great pleasure.
Dried herbs are good to use, but fresh is always best. Below are a few
varieties of herbs that are easy to grow:

      Parsley - curly leaf and continental are both very easy to grow,
      Basil - vietnamese, thai and bush basil are all delicious
      Chives - garlic and plain
      Garlic - standard or elephant (milder)
      Lemongrass
      Rosemary
      Coriander - vietnamese and standard
      Sage
      Oregano
      Dill and Fennel
      Mint

If you do not have enough ground area, most herbs grow well and look
great in pots and hanging baskets. This is a good idea if you live in an
apartment or unit and only have a porch or balcony.

Lemongrass is a reed and grows well in a rockery or pot. Mature leaves can
be used whole in cooking, then removed before serving or brewed in boiling
water for tea - bulbs can be chopped finely or crushed with a tenderiser
mallet and used for cooking.

Mint needs to be contained in a pot or basket as roots spread rapidly.
Good mint varieties are;
    Spearmint - strong, rich sharp flavour, refreshing aroma.
    Peppermint - stronger than spearmint, hotter flavour, more pungent.
    Apple mint - smaller softer leaf, milder more subtle flavour, definite apple
    smell- comes in plain green or green/cream variegated leaf.
    Chocolate mint - is great for desserts and grows well in hanging baskets.

All varieties of parsley do well in pots, grow 2 or 3 varieties. They also look
attractive in a rockery or cottage garden.

Sage also looks good in these areas. Pineapple sage is very attractive and
bears bright green leaves with red sprays of small flowers. It is very tasty

chopped into salads, stir fries, sweet and sour dishes, savoury muffins, omelettes and quiches. It is best to use the young tender leaves.

RECIPE TIPS:
Ingredients such as flour, vegetables, fruits, nuts, lentils or liquids can be substituted, as long as they make up the same amounts as stated in the recipes. Herbs and seasonings should be used to individual taste and may be adjusted before serving.

Many of these recipes are designed for more than one person. You can halve or double the ingredients if needed.

Now start preparing and good luck. I know you will be rewarded for your time when you taste these delicious, healthy and satisfying liver friendly foods.

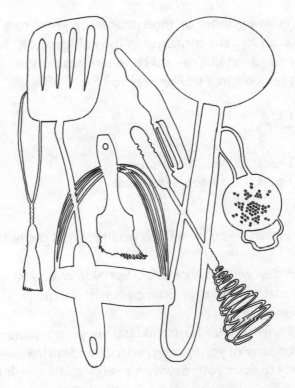

Linseed

Much has been written about the benefits of linseed (flaxseed) in our diets and we now find it in many of our bread and cereal products. Since the introduction of LSA - linseed, sunflower seed and almonds some time ago, many of us have added this mixture to our favourite recipes such as drinks, cereals, soups, dips, casseroles, cakes, biscuits, desserts, in fact anything which can include a meal substance. LSA is an excellent source of healthy fatty acids, protein, calcium, phosphorus, potassium, iron, magnesium, copper, manganese, selenium, vitamin A, vitamin E and B group vitamins .

Now we have LAA - Linseed, Alfalfa seed and Almonds. So, as well as all the above mentioned nutritional benefits, alfalfa seeds will provide plant hormones, chlorophyll (a natural cleanser) and many of the essential vitamins and minerals.

LAA

4 tbsp	linseeds
I tbsp	alfalfa seeds
3 tbsp	almonds

Use a coffee grinder or food processor, grind to a fine meal
Store in an airtight container in the refrigerator,
Use as required but re-seal to retain freshness.
Use in recipes, in a similar way to LSA

LSA

I cup	almonds
2 cups	sunflower seeds
3 cups	linseeds (flaxseeds)

Please note that if you have Diverticulitis, grind the nuts and seeds first.

Start your day with LSA or LAA. Sprinkle over your usual cereal, on sandwiches, toast, muffins or crumpets with tahini, jam or nut paste (no butter or margarine).
If you only like fresh fruit for breakfast, chop up a banana, some melon, strawberries or any of your preferred fruit and sprinkle with LSA or LAA. This is the way to start your day with energy and avoid hunger until lunch time.

We can show you that just by using liver friendly foods and taking a little time to select recipes to suit your food tolerance, you will soon hear friends say,

"Gee! you look well, you are lucky to be so healthy"
Luck has nothing to do with it!

Being healthy and looking good, is to do with you taking control of your own lifestyle and eating foods to help your liver perform its cleansing function. Note the foods to which you are intolerant, and adjust your meals accordingly.

A tip to get you through that between - meals - hunger - boredom- and cravings time - fill 2 x 1 litre carafes with drinking water, place one in the kitchen and one in your work space. If you find it difficult to drink lots of water remember small quantities often, will soon get you in the habit of drinking more water. Try to drink water in between meals - this goes for tea and coffee as well.

Every night prepare a platter of bite size snacks. Place it centre front top shelf of the refrigerator, so that it is easily seen when you are looking for nibbles.

Carrot and celery sticks, snow peas, cauliflower florets and any other vegetable you like raw, a couple of pieces of fruit, grapes and small wedges of melon, some dried fruits and nuts. You cannot eat it all in one day and the variety will make you feel that you are not deprived of snacks. This will stop you from grazing on the wrong foods. Allow yourself no more than 3 - 4 of these snacks a day.

If friends pop in for tea or coffee offer a sweet treat. Have some treats on hand made from the recipes in this book

Any vegetable pieces left over from your platter can be used in a salad or your evening meal. Fruits can be made into a fruit salad for dessert.

Keep the Platter, Simple, Varied and Fresh!

AUDREY TEA HINT:

Recipes of all kinds are simply a list of ingredients combined together to attain a certain flavour and texture. A recipe is a guidline - the cook can substitute, experiment with new things, change ingredients to taste, while keeping within the guidelines. The result will often be magical!

beverages

juices galore - another great start! ♥

If you have a juice extractor, do yourself a favour and try different combinations. Fruits and vegetables juiced together taste fantastic. Some simple combinations are;

1. carrot, fresh ginger, apple
2. carrot, celery, parsley, mint, tomato, apple
3. beetroot, apple, pear, ginger, parsley
4. orange, lemon (whole), carrot, fresh ginger, parsley

fruity energiser drink ♥

1	yellow pear skin on, core removed
1	granny smith apple skin on, core removed
1/2 cup	oat, soy, rice or almond milk
1 tsp	honey
1 scoop	vitari ice cream
4	mint leaves

Mix in food processor until smooth.
Add sprinkle of cinnamon.

Any combination of fruit is great and you may try juices of peaches, pineapples, nectarines, passionfruits or plums, just to name a few.

AUDREY TEA HINT
All juices are best if they are processed as you need them.
Store in the refrigerator for up to 24 hours.
Always rinse the juice extractor immediately after each use.

chlorophyll hit

2	carrots, tops removed
3	beetroot tops
1 cup	parsley tops, chopped
3	spinach leaves
1 small	apple seeded

Pass all through the juicer and serve with crushed ice

garlic cleanser

1 cup	parsley tops chopped
1-3 cloves	garlic
2	carrots, tops removed
2 stalks	celery

Pass all through the juicer and add a squeeze of fresh lemon

liver purifier

2 large	spinach leaves
3	broccoli flowerets
1-2 cloves	garlic
1	green pepper
1 cup	parsley tops, chopped
1	red apple, seeded

Pass all through a juicer,
This juice is great to add your liver tonic powder to.
High in vitamin C and sulphur compounds to cleanse the liver!

Doing the best you can, makes you the hero of your own story. Audrey Tea

tropical cocktail

1	apple seeded
1 cup	coconut milk
1 wedge	fresh pineapple (4 inches/10cm)

Pass apple and pineapple through juicer, pour juice into a glass
Add coconut milk. Stir well.
Serve with crushed ice and a wedge of pineapple.
Fantastic for a summer breakfast.

tomato spice

2	red tomatoes
1	red pepper
1 cup	parsley tops, chopped
1 large	spinach leaf
1 dash	Tabasco sauce (if desired)
1 pinch	tumeric powder (if desired)

Pass vegetables through juicer and add Tabasco and tumeric and mix in.
This is energising and cleansing.

digestive tonic juice

1	beetroot
1 piece	fresh ginger root (about 1 inch/2.5cm)
1/2	red apple seeded
1	carrot, tops removed
	Large slice papaya

Pass through the juicer.
This juice aids digestion and is healing and soothing for the stomach.
For digestive problems - mix in 1-teaspoon of slippery elm powder.

dynamic lifter

1	pear
1	banana
1 cup	rice, oat or soy milk
1	prune
2 tbsp	LSA
2	dates
1/4 cup	orange juice

Mix in blender or food processor until smooth.

banana heaven

2	bananas
1 cup	rice, oat or soy milk
4	dates
2 tbsp	LSA

Mix in blender or food processor until smooth.

summer tang

1/2 punnet	raspberries
1 peeled	kiwi Fruit
1/2 cup	lemon juice
1	banana
1 tbsp	LSA
1/2 cup	orange juice

Mix in blender or food processor until smooth.
Add some crushed ice and bingo you have a mock cocktail.

We can do no great things, only small things, with GREAT love.
Mother Theresa

mint tea

2 tbsp	chinese green tea
4 tbsp	spearmint (or mint) chopped
900ml/32oz	water
4 slices	lemon thinly sliced
Honey to taste	
Extra mint for garnish	

Add tea and mint to a teapot.
Boil the water then pour into pot.
Leave for 5 minutes.
Pour the tea through a strainer into warmed glasses.
Add honey to taste and a slice of lemon.
Add sprig of mint for garnish.
Can be served hot or cold, poured over ice. Delicious!

berry shake

I cup	berries (variety)
I tsp	coriander finely diced
I cup	almond, rice or oat milk
I tbsp	maple syrup or honey
2 tblsp	LSA
I tsp	orange rind grated

Blend all the ingredients together and serve

To achieve the impossible you must first attempt the difficult.
Audrey Tea

spiced tea

6	cloves, whole
2 strips	lemon rind
I stick	cinnamon bark
2 tsp	tea (Formosan is yum)
2 tbsp	ginger grated
5	lemon rings to serve

Bring 5 cups of water, lemon rind, cloves, cinnamon and ginger to the boil.
Simmer for 10 minutes, then return to the boil.
Pour the mixture into a teapot with the tea.
Leave for a couple of minutes.
Strain and serve with lemon rind.
Honey is optional

mover and shaker

I clove	garlic
I	lemon, whole
3	carrots
2 sticks	celery
I bunch	parsley
I small	beetroot
I	apple
4	spinach leaves

Place all ingredients into juicer.
Drink immediately and wait for the buzz!

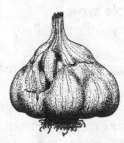

breakfasts

sweet rice porridge

serves 2

I cup	rice basmati/jasmin/brown, cooked, keep warm
I tsp	honey (optional)
2 tsp	LSA
I sprinkle	sultanas
2 tbsp	papya or paw paw
1/2 cup	oat, soy or rice milk, warmed

Put soy milk, sultanas and honey into a saucepan and heat.
Put the warm rice into a breakfast bowl.
Cut the fruit into bite size cubes and put on the rice.
Pour on the heated soy milik.
Sprinkle with LSA.

wild about berries ❤

serves 4 or more

I cup	raspberries, fresh
I cup	blueberries fresh
I cup	boysenberries, fresh
I cup	strawberries, fresh
I cup	mulberries or raspberries - place in freezer
1/4 cup	maple syrup
300ml(10oz)	soy yoghurt (chilled)

Trim berries and slice strawberries, add maple syrup, toss gently
Place in individual serving comports.
Just before serving, whiz the yoghurt and frozen berries together to
make whipped type of soft ice confection.
Serve and garnish with chopped mint.

muesli with the lot ♥

Natural sweetness of the fruit makes this delicious

2 cups	rolled oats
2 cups	processed bran (allbran)
1 cup	oat bran
1 cup	rice bran
1 cup	natural sultanas
1 cup	currants
1/2 cup	dried apricots, chopped
1/2 cup	almonds, chopped
1/2 cup	pumpkin seeds
1/2 cup	sunflower seeds

Mix all together, store in an air tight container away from light
One serve = 3 - 4 tablespoons muesli + oat, soy or rice milk
       +1 dstsp LSA + 1 teaspoon lecithin.

AUDREY TEA HINT
A large quantity of muesli can be made. Store it in an airtight container, in the refrigerator. Sticky tape some bay leaves on the inside of the lid.

charles's poached eggs

serves 1

2 large	eggs, poached in simmering water
2 thick slices	dark rye, toasted
1	tomato, cut in half
1 tbsp	tahini
1 clove	garlic, thinly sliced (optional)
lashings of LSA	
salt and ground black pepper to taste	

Toast bread and spread with tahini, thickly. The garlic goes next.
Place poached eggs on toast and tomatoes next to toast
Sprinkle heavily with LSA and garnish with parsley. Yum!

muffins for weekend brunch ❤

approx 12 muffins

I large	egg
1/2 cup	soy milk
2 tbsp	cold pressed olive oil
I tbsp	honey
I cup	wholemeal SR flour
I tbsp	LSA

Place egg, milk and oil in a bowl and whisk with fork.
Place flour in large bowl, make a well in middle and pour in liquid then honey.
Mix lightly, do not overstir.
Place mixture in greased muffin tins,
Sprinkle tops lightly with cinnamon and sesame seeds.

variations

apricot
add;

I tbsp	soy yoghurt to liquid
1/2 cup	dried apricots, chopped
2 tbsp	shredded coconut.

apple
add;

I	apple, grated skin on
1/2 cup	sultanas
I tsp	cinnamon to dry ingredients before mixing liquid.

banana
add

I	banana, mashed
1/2 cup	walnuts to mixture.

top with extra nuts or sunflower seeds.

All variations are delicious served with a pile of berries on the side

buckwheat pancakes

makes approx 12 med pancakes

Use a non-stick fry pan for this recipe
The pancakes can be either like pikelets or thin crepes

1 cup	buckwheat flour
1	egg
1/2 cup	rice milk (or more)

Place flour into mixing bowl
Add egg
Pour in rice milk, half a cup first, stir
Keep adding milk and whisking until the texture is heavy, but firm - like stiff cream
Pour mixture into a hot frypan
Cook until golden on either side
Make a stack, cover with either honey and lemon, maple syrup, a mixture of berries or poached eggs.

sweet rhubarb porridge

serves 2 or more

Delicious for breakfast or sweets

1 cup	jasmin or basmati rice washed
1 cup	rhubarb
1/2 cup	coconut cream
rice syrup as needed	

Wash the rice thoroughly before cooking, it makes it light and fluffy.
Cook rice until soft, drain and rinse under cold water
Put cooked rhubarb, rice syrup and half the coconut cream in a food processor and blend.
Pour blended mixture over rice.

Serve chilled with a teaspoon of coconut cream and a sprig of mint

something light for breakfast ❤

Toast some thick slices of bread - grainy, light rye or sour dough
Spread with tahini.
Sprinkle with LSA, chopped nuts or currants and natural sultanas and a
few sesame seeds.
Pop under the griller, long enough to just warm the topping.

banana crepes

approx 12 or more crepes

Use a non-stick fry pan for this recipe, make the pancakes thin.

1 cup	buckwheat flour
1	egg
1/2 cup	oat or rice milk (or more)
2 ripe	bananas

Place flour into mixing bowl, add egg,
Pour in rice milk, half a cup first, stir if needed add more
Mash banana and add to mixture.
Add remaining milk and whisk until the texture is like heavy, but runny.
Pour mixture into a hot frypan, cook until golden on either side

sardines on toast

1 tin	sardines
1	lemon, juiced
1 tbsp	tahini
1 clove	garlic, crushed
1	tomato, sliced
2 pieces	rice bread
salt and ground black pepper to taste	

Put sardines, lemon juice and garlic in a bowl, mash up with a fork
Toast bread, spread with tahini, put on sardine mixture
Add tomato on top of sardines.

hot, healthy and hearty porridge ♥

serves 2 - 3

1/2 cup	rolled oats
1/2 cup	oat bran
1/2 cup	rice bran
1/2 cup	natural raisins
1 dsp	lecithin granules (optional)
1 tbsp	LSA
3/4 cup	water
1/2 cup	oat or soy milk

Soak dry ingredients overnight in water, then drain liquid.
Combine water and soy milk, add to mixture
Cook for 5 minutes, stir often.
Add more soy milk until you get the consistency you prefer.

Serve with a few pitted prunes or drained cooked apricots.

poached fruit

serves 2 - 3

6 small	pears
2 strips	lemon peel, use a peeler
2 tbsp	pear concentrate (sweetener)
1 cup	water

Use a stainless steel or ceramic bowl
Fill saucepan 1/4 full of water and place bowl on top
Peel pears (any fruit will taste fantastic) and place in bowl
Place lemon peel, water and pear concentrate with pears
Experiment with the sweetness that best suits your taste buds
The water in the saucepan will boil and the steam heats the bowl
When the fruit is cooked, let cool. Will store in the refrigerator.

AUDREY TEA HINT
Never be intimidated by a long list of ingredients!

the big breakfast

For Sunday mornings or times of need.

2 large	eggs, poached
1	tomato, halved and grilled
1 cup	field and button mushrooms, grilled
1 stack	buckwheat pancakes (see page 177)
	cold pressed olive oil
	maple syrup for pouring (optional)
	parsley for garnish

Have a warm stack of buckwheat pancakes in the oven
Poach the eggs, grill the tomatoes
Wash the mushrooms and drizzle with oil,
Leave them as whole, place mushrooms under griller
Place 2 pankaces on a plate, pile on eggs, tomatoes, mushrooms
Drizzle on the maple syrup and garnish with parsley

Serve with a big raw vegetable juice

fruit salad ❤

serves 2 or more

1	apple, cut into bite size pieces
1	pear, cut into bite size pieces
2	nectarine, cut into bite size pieces
1/4	rockmelon, cut into bite size pieces
1 punnet	strawberries, sliced in half
1/2 cup	cashews and Brazil nuts, crushed up
handful	sultanas or raisins
1	lemon, juiced
	maple syrup and LSA

Combine all ingredients, add lashings of LSA and serve

soups

tasty chunky tomato lentil soup ❤

serves 6- 8

Suitable to freeze in meal size portions
This soup can be served chunky or if preferred smooth,
For a smooth soup, pureé with a hand held food processor.

810g/29oz	tomatoes, chopped, tin
I cup	red lentils (soaked for I hour)
2 cups	boiling water
I cup	celery, chopped
I tbsp	garlic, chopped
I tbsp	basil leaves, chopped fresh
1/2 cup	parsley, chopped
I large	onion, chopped
I tbsp	lemon juice
1/2 tsp	rock salt
1/2 tsp	pepper, freshly ground
I tbsp	tomato paste (or more)
I dstsp	cold pressed olive oil

(garlic and basil according to your personal taste)

Pour the boiling water over the lentils and soak for I hour
Brown onion and garlic in oil in a non stick pan
Add to other ingredients in a large pan.
Simmer gently until all is tender, approx I hour.
Add more water if necessary.
Season to taste

Serve sprinkled with chopped parsley.

spinach soup

serves 6

This soup can be served chunky.
For a smooth soup, pureé with a hand held food processor.

2 bunches	spinach, washed and heavy stems taken out
4 large	potatoes
4 cups	stock, vegetable or chicken
I cup	water
I	onion
2 cloves	garlic, crushed
I	lemon, juiced

salt and ground black pepper to taste
cold pressed olive oil

Brown onion and garlic in oil in a saucepan
Peel and cut the potato into chunks
Add the potato to onion and brown
Add stock and water and simmer gently until all is tender
Add chopped spinach
Season to taste
If you would like to have a smooth soup - purée now

Serve with a vegetable salad and bread

SOUP LOVERS
A tip for soup lovers is to roast your vegetables in the oven first, as it brings
out the flavour. Then place them in the saucepan and continue as per recipe.

fish and garlic soup

serves 6 - 8

Any fish and/or your favourite shellfish can be used for this soup

2 sticks	celery, sliced
2 large	potatoes, chopped (peeled if desired)
1 whole	chilli, seeded, sliced (optional)
4+1/2 cups	stock, fish or vegetable
2 kg (4.4lbs)	fish and shellfish prepared
2	onions, chopped
10 cloves	garlic, half thinly sliced, half crushed
6 med	tomatoes, ripe, chopped
1 bunch	dill, chopped
1 bunch	parsley, chopped
1 bunch	coriander
2	lemon, juiced
3 tbsp	cold pressed olive oil

salt and ground black pepper to taste

Brown onion, thinly sliced garlic and celery in oil for 2 minutes
Add the crushed garlic and chilli, cook for 1 minute
Add potaotes, stir constantly till slightly golden
Pour in stock and lemon juice
Simmer until potatoes are tender
Add fish, shell fish, tomatoes, herbs and seasoning
Cook gently until seafood is tender

Serve with a vegetable salad and crusty bread

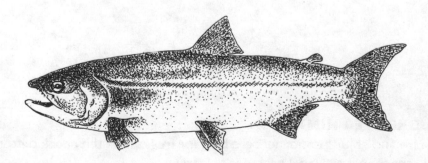

fresh vegetable consomme ❤

serves 6

1 tbsp	whole black peppercorns
4 cloves	garlic
2	bay leaves

tie the above three ingredients into a muslin bag

1 + 1/2L /50oz	water
3 stalks	celery
2 large	carrots
1 med	leek, wash and thinly sliced into rings
1 med	parsnip
220g/8oz	broccoli, small florets
1 dstsp	cold pressed olive oil
1 dstsp	tomato paste

Cut carrot and celery into small thin strips
Brown leeks in hot oil in large saucepan
Add all other ingredients except broccoli
Simmer for about 15 minutes
Discard muslin bag, add broccoli and continue to simmer a further 5 minutes
Sprinkle with chopped parsley when serving, season to taste

AUDREY TEA HINT
Square and oblong containers are best for freezing as they pack better and save space. Always label each pack clearly.

potato and leek soup ♥

serves 6

750g /27oz	potatoes, peeled,chopped
I large	leek, washed and sliced
I med	white radish, chopped
I tbsp	garlic, chopped
1/2 tsp	dry mustard
1/2 tsp	curry powder
I cup	soy or rice milk

sea salt and cracked pepper to taste

Place all ingredients in a large pan, barely cover with water
Gently simmer with the lid on until tender, approx 30 - 40 minutes
Pureé in blender while adding milk until smooth

Serve with a sprinkle of paprika and fingers of grain bread

roast tomato soup

serves 6

4 cups	very ripe tomatoes, chopped
I large	onion
4 cloves	garlic
2 large	potatoes, chopped
3 tbsp	cold pressed olive oil
2 cups	vegetable stock

sea salt and cracked pepper to taste

Place all ingredients in baking pan
Bake in very hot oven until cooked
Put all the ingredients into a saucepan and purée
Heat slightly and serve

green and white soup ❤

serves 8 - 10

Suitable to freeze.
Great as a chunky soup but if preferred creamy, add 2 cups soy milk and pureé with blender.

5	spring onions, tops chopped
1 cup	celery, chopped
1 cup	parsley, chopped
1 cup	broccoli florets, small
1 cup	cauliflower florets, small
1 cup	green beans, cut small
1 cup	green cabbage, finely chopped
1 cup	parsnip, grated
1 cup	potato, grated
2 small	green whole chilli (optional)
1 tbsp	garlic, chopped (optional)
1 tsp	lemon juice
1/2 cup	green capsicum, chopped

cracked pepper and sea salt to taste

Place all ingredients in a large pan
Add enough water to barely cover vegetables
Simmer until tender, approx 1 hour
Taste and season if necessary

Garnish with chopped spring onion tops

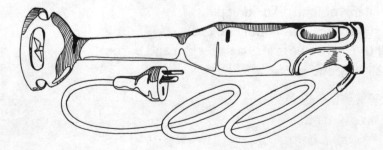

chicken and vegetable noodle soup ❤

serves 6 - 8

Suitable to freeze in serving portions.

4	chicken drumsticks, skinned
2 cups	carrot, grated
I cup	parsnip, grated
I cup	swede, grated
I cup	celery, chopped
1/2 cup	parsley, chopped
I medium	onion, chopped, browned in pan
2 cups	egg noodles, slightly crushed
I can	whole corn, including liquid
5 cups	water or vegetable stock
cold pressed olive oil	

Brown onion in the saucepan with oil
Place all other ingredients in the saucepan
Simmer for about an hour until tender.
Remove chicken bones leaving meat in soup
Season with black pepper and rock salt to taste.

pumpkin soup ❤

serves 6

500g/18oz	pumpkin, peeled chunks
125g/4-5oz	potato, peeled chunks
I large	onion, thinly sliced
I cup	chicken or vegetable stock
1/2 cup	parsley chopped
sea salt and cracked pepper to taste	

Place all ingredients in large pan barely covering with water
Simmer until tender with the lid on for approx. 30 - 45 minutes
Season to taste before blending to a puree

Serve with a sprinkle of ground nutmeg and garnish with chopped parsley

green lentil, leek and spinach soup

serves 4 or more

This soup is full of goodness and revives the senses, its great in summer or winter with crusty bread.
This soup can be made with chicken, or vegetable stock.

350g/12oz	green lentils (cover with water for two hours)
3	leeks, finely chopped
3 cloves	garlic, crushed
3 large	potatoes, peeled and chopped into bite size chunks
3	bay leaves
1 tsp	oregano
1/2 tsp	thyme
1/3 cup	lemon juice
4 cups	vegetable stock
8 cups	water
500g/18oz	spinach, washed, heavy stems removed, chopped
cold pressed olive oil	
sea salt and cracked pepper to taste	

Heat in a heavy saucepan and add oil
Add garlic and leeks, cook for two minutes
Add potatoes and cook for a further three minutes
Add thyme, oregano, stock, water and drained lentils
Simmer for 40 minutes
Stir occassionally
When lentils are tender, grind black pepper and stir in lemon juice and spinach
Cook for another two minutes

Serve with fresh bread

potato and sweetcorn chowder ❤

serves 4 or more

1 large	potato, peeled and chopped
2 sticks	celery, finely sliced
1 large	onion, chopped
600ml/20oz	chicken or vegetable stock
300ml/10oz	soy or rice milk
2 cloves	garlic, crushed
2 tbsp	cold pressed olive oil
250g/9oz tin	butter beans, drained and rinsed
300g/11oz	corn kernels scraped off the cob or canned
1/4 tsp	thyme or sage
2 tbsp	chopped parsley
sea salt and cracked pepper to taste	

In a large saucepan, brown onion and garlic for two minutes
Add potato and celery
Turn down the heat
Stir often with a wooden spoon for another two minutes
Stir in stock and cover pan
Simmer gently for 20 minutes
Add corn, beans, milk and sage
Season with pepper and salt

Serve sprinkled with parsley and crusty bread.

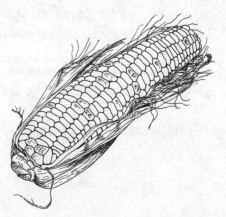

dips, spreads, dressings

salmon or tuna dips ❤

210g/7-8oz	pink salmon, tin
2 tbsp	tofu (fresh bean curd) crumbled or grated
1 med	onion, finely chopped
2 tbsp	carrot grated
2 tbsp	parsley, chopped
1 pinch	chilli powder (optional)

Mash fish and bones with a fork.
Mix in all other ingredients using enough of the fish juices to make a blended spread.
Add a squeeze of lemon juice and salt and pepper to taste.

piquant fresh herb dip ❤

1 cup	natural soy yoghurt
1 tbsp	basil, chopped
1 tbsp	parsley, chopped
1 tbsp	chives, chopped
1 tbsp	tomato paste
1 tsp	dijon mustard
2 large	garlic cloves, crushed
1/2 tsp	cracked black pepper

Combine all ingredients and mix well.
Chill in refrigerator for a couple of hours to allow flavours to blend

Serve garnished with chopped parsley.

hoummus

400g/14oz	chickpeas, drained and rinsed (canned or cooked)
3 tbsp	tahini
1 clove	garlic, crushed (more if desired)
2	lemons juiced

Mix all together in a blender

broadbean dip

500g/18oz	broadbeans, frozen or fresh
1 tsp	cummin powder
1 tsp	cardamon powder
2 cloves	garlic, crushed (more if desired)
1	lemon juiced
1 whole	chilli, seeded and diced (optional)

Cook beans in water with cummin, cardamon and garlic.
Drain beans and retain juice
Add lemon juice and retrieve the garlic, place with the beans
Purée all together - add more juice if necessary

Serve warm with vegetable sticks or cold with crackers or on sandwiches.

dressing no 1 ❤

1 cup	cold pressed sesame oil
1 tbsp	fresh garlic, crushed
1/2 cup	lemon juice
1/2 tsp	cumin, dried
1	lemon, juiced

Put all ingredients into a jar, shake until well mixed.
Store in refrigerator.

dressing no 2 ❤

1/2 cup	balsamic vinegar or lemon juice
1/2 cup	cold pressed olive oil
1 dstsp	tamari
1 tsp	mixed herbs

Put all ingredients into a jar, shake well until mixed,
Store in refrigerator.

dressing no 3 ❤

1/2 cup	natural soy yoghurt
1/2 cup	lemon or orange juice
1 tbsp	mint, chopped

Mix only as required.

dressing no 4

2	lemons juiced
3 tbsp	hoummus
1 clove	garlic, crushed
1 tbsp	cold pressed olive oil (optional)

Mix all together in a jar

dressing no 5

1 tbsp	honey
2 tsp	grainy mustard
2 - 3 tbsp	cold pressed olive oil (optional)
2	lemons, juiced

Mix all together in a jar

salads, sides and snacks

sprouts, sprouts and more sprouts

There are some wonderful varieties of fresh sprouts - try a different one each week. Loosely separate the sprouts and gently toss together. Include one of the hotter varieties such as radish or mustard sprouts, and add just a little lemon juice to your taste. Prepare just the amount you need as this sprout salad is best eaten fresh.

NOTE: Remaining sprouts will store well in the fridge in the plastic containers in which they were packed and sold.

Salads are a mixture of fruits and vegetables so try a few mixtures of your own choice. Salads do not have to have a dressing and many people prefer salads without dressing. If you are using ingredients that turn brown after they are cut, then you need to toss them in lemon juice, to stop this discolouration.

salad garnishes
vegetable waves
Using a vegetable peeler carefully slice down the length of vegetables such as carrots, lebanese cucumbers, red and white radishes, zucchinis etc, so that you have long thin slices the length of your vegetable.
Vegetables such as carrots and radishes can be placed in really cold water for up to 30 minutes before use for extra crispness.

vegetable curls
Cut sticks of vegetable about 6 cm long, cut 2 or 3 slits with a sharp knife into one end of each piece, stand in cold water in fridge for an hour and the end will curl - celery, carrot and radish are great for this.

vegetable strings
Push grater lengthways down vegetable to get long thin strings. Use crisp vegetables such as carrot, radish, beetroot and Japanese pumpkin.

beetroot and coriander salad

serves 3

1 bunch	coriander
2 med	beetroots, washed and peeled
4 tbsp	lemon or lime juice
4 tbsp	LSA
2 tbsp	sunflower seeds, dry roasted
2	carrots, grated

Wash and dice the coriander.
Wash and peel the beets and carrots
Grate carrots and the beets. Be careful as the red juice gets everywhere!
Put into a salad bowl, put in the LSA.
To roast the seeds -
Heat a small pan, add the sunflowers. Keep them moving.
When they turn golden brown, take them off the heat.
Pour the lemon juice over the salad.
Then toss on the hot sizzling sunflower seeds.

gourmet golden pumpkins ❤

serves 6

2 to 4	golden nugget or butternut pumpkins
4 cloves	garlic, crushed
1 med	onion, diced or 4 spring onions, chopped
1 + 1/2 cups	brown rice, cooked
1/4 tsp	coriander, ground
1/4 tsp	cumin, ground
1 pinch	nutmeg
2 tsp	shoyu or tamari

Cut small top off pumpkin and scoop out seeds, replace top
Bake in moderate oven for 30 minutes, until tender.
Cool slightly and scrape out cooked pumpkin flesh from shell
Take care not to damage the shell. Mix pumpkin and all other ingredients
together - spoon back into the shell.
Drizzle a little sweet chilli sauce on top of mixture (optional)

hot, crisp and mellow salad ❤

serves 4 - 6

15 small	radishes
1	green apple, cored, quartered, thinly sliced
1 small	mango, peeled and sliced
2 stalks	celery, thinly sliced
1/2 cup	walnuts, chopped

dressing

1/2 cup	natural soy yoghurt
1 dstsp	horseradish sauce
1 tbsp	dill, freshly chopped

salt and ground black pepper
dill for garnish

Top and tail radishes, slice thinly.
Add to dressing with thinly sliced apple and celery and walnuts
Peel, stone and cube mango, fold into mixture
Garnish with dill

Served chilled in a bowl

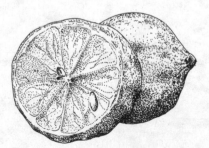

corn and carrot salad ♥

serves 4

2 med	carrots, peeled
2	corn cobs
2 med	potatoes, peeled
3 tbsp	sunflower seeds, dry roasted
2 small	sweet potatoes, peeled

dressing

2	garlic cloves, crushed
2 tbsp	lemon juice
1 tbsp	tamari
1 tbsp	tahini

Wash and peel all the vegetables
Cut all vegetables into bite sized pieces
Peel the corn and cut into thick rings
Put all the vegetables into a steamer and cook until tender
Don't over cook them. Let cool and add the sunflower seeds

For the dressing, mix all the ingredients together.
If it becomes too thick because of the tahini, add a small amount of
water or lemon juice

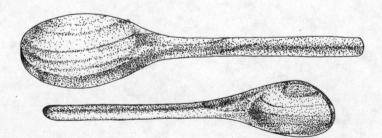

big green salad

serves 4 - 6

Experiment with any other green vegetable you like.

I bunch	English spinach, washed & torn
2 cups	snow peas, stringed
2 cups	broccoli, florets
2 bunches	asparagus
I cup	basil and parsley, chopped
2 med	lebanese cucumbers, thin strips
I med	capsicum green, seeded, sliced
I cup	green beans, cut in half
4 tbsp	LSA

Wash all the vegetables
Cut the tough ends off the asparagus and discard
Put the broccoli, asparagus and beans into a steamer, cook until tender
Don't over cook them
Tear up the lettuce and spinach and put into a large salad bowl
Put the snowpeas, capsicum and all the cooked vegetables into the bowl
Toss in the herbs

Serve with a dressing of your choice
Or with lemon and cold pressed olive oil poured over the top.

nice cool salad ❤

To serve as a side dish with spicy foods

2	lebanese cucumbers
I large	carrot
I tbsp	mint, chopped
1/2 cup	natural soy yoghurt, chilled

Grate cucumbers and carrot
Combine all ingredients

avocado a light start entree ❤

serves 4

2 large	avocados
125g/4-5oz	pink salmon, tin
1 dstsp	tomato paste
2	spring onions, tops finely chopped
1	lemon juiced
1 tbsp	soft tofu

Tabasco sauce to taste
ground black pepper to taste

Cut avocados in half lengthways. scoop all flesh and mash into a bowl.
Mash drained fish and bones
Add mashed avocados with all other ingredients until evenly mixed.
Add a little of fish juice if necessary for smooth mix.
Taste and add more seasoning if necessary.
Fill avocado shells with mixture.

Serve individually and garnish with slice of cucumber, tomato and alfalfa sprouts.

Use leftovers as a dip or sandwich spread.

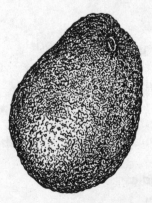

savoury hash browns ❤

6 - 12 hash browns

4 tbsp	cold pressed olive oil
500g/18oz	potatoes, lightly cooked and grated
1	onion, finely chopped
1 tbsp	mint, chopped
1	egg, beaten
salt and black pepper to taste	

Mix all ingredients together, except oil
Heat oil in a large pan, when hot add potato mixture
Press flat and cook on moderate heat till golden brown, flip till golden
Repeat till all the mixture is gone

Serve anytime for, breakfast, snack, or as a side with meal

anytime quick vegetables ❤

4 or more

1/4	cabbage, sliced
1 dsp	cold pressed sesame seed oil
1 tsp	ginger, grated
1/2 cup	bamboo shoots
1/2 cup	bean shoots
125g/4-5oz	snow peas
100g/3-4oz	field mushrooms
1/2 cup	water
1 dstsp	tamari
2 cups	chinese noodles (ready to eat)
cold pressed olive oil	

Sautè ginger in oil in a large pan or wok
Add cabbage and cook for 2 minutes tossing all the time.
Add all other vegetables and cook another 2 minutes.
Add to mixture with noodles, tossing all the time until all heated through.

Serve as a snack or side vegetable or cold as a salad.

pumpkin piquant salad ❤

serves 6

1 cup	blue pumpkin, grated or in thin strips
4	spring onions, thinly sliced diagonally
1/2 cup	raisins
1/2 cup	walnuts or pecan pieces
1 tbsp	fennel - fresh, thinly sliced
1 med	orange, peeled and cut into chunks
1 tbsp	mint, chopped
1 tbsp	lemon juice
1 clove	garlic, crushed

Mix all together, cover and stand in refrigerater for about an hour
Serve with dressing no 1(see page 191)

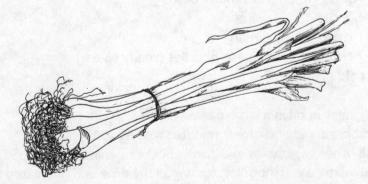

mixed vegetable salad ❤

4 or more

1 large	carrot, cut into thin strips
200g/7oz	broccoli florets
300g/11oz	cauliflower florets
2 sticks	celery, cut into thin slices
400g/14oz	berlotti beans, drained/rinsed
6 baby	potatoes, steamed
400g/14oz	lentils, drained and halved
1 small	red capsicum
2 tbsp	garlic chives fresh, chopped
2 tbsp	oregano, chopped
2 tbsp	parsley, chopped
2 tbsp	mint, chopped
4	hard boiled eggs chopped
10	snow peas, trimmed
3/4 cup	no 1 dressing

Steam carrot, broccoli and cauliflower until cooked but still crisp.
Cool and mix all other ingredients together except the dressing.
Cover in bowl and refrigerate overnight.
Fold dressing through before serving.

Serve with your favourite bread or a bowl of delicious roast vegetables

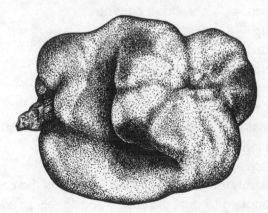

sweet savoury salad ❤

4 or more

1 cup	watermelon, balled or diced
1 cup	cantaloupe (rock melon) balled or diced
1 cup	honey-dew melon, balled or diced
1 cup	mint, chopped or if you prefer parsley
1/2 cup	pumpkin seeds
1/4 cup	toasted sesame seeds
1/4 cup	lemon or orange juice

Mix all ingredients gently together
Let stand in refrigerator, in an airtight container for 1/2 hour to allow flavours to blend

Serve individually in small lettuce cups on a large platter

savoury banana salad ❤

4 or more

Tasty salad served with crumbed fish, curries and chicken dishes
Store in refrigerator in airtight container

2 large	bananas, firm ripe
1 large	red apple
1/2 cup	shredded coconut
1/2 cup	roasted cashews
1/2 cup	soy natural yoghurt
1/4 cup	light malt vinegar
1/4 cup	orange juice, fresh

Mix the dressing of yoghurt, vinegar and juice in a large bowl
Slice the banana
Core and dice apple, leave skin
Toss immediately into dressing, blend in most of the coconut and cashews
Leave just enough to dust the top of this lovely salad

fresh and corny ❤

serves 4 - 6

2 cups	corn niblets, fresh, young and juicy
1 large	red apple
2 tbsp	mint, fresh, chopped
4	spring onions, thinly sliced
1	naval orange, peeled of all pith and cubed
1 large	lemon, juiced
ground black pepper to taste	

Take leaves and fibres from corn cobs
Use a sharp knife remove corn niblets carefully, keep the niblets whole
Core and dice apple leaving skin, toss immediately into lemon juice
Mix all ingredients together and serve

refreshing cucumber salad ❤

4 or more

4 small	cucumbers, lebanese or small continental
1	red onion, finely chopped
1 tbsp	mint, chopped fresh
1 small	green capsicum, thinly sliced
1/2 cup	tarragon vinegar
sea salt and ground black pepper to taste	

Wash cucumbers, score skins with a fork, rinse then slice thinly
Mix all ingredients and toss together

The purpose of life is to discover your gifts. The meaning of life is to give your gifts away with love.

greens 'n' things ♥

serves 6 - 8

I cup	broccoli florets
I cup	celery, diced
I cup	green capsicum, diced
I cup	green beans, chopped
6	spring onions, tops and all chopped
I cup	snow peas, trimmed
I cup	parsley, chopped
I cup	cucumber, lebanese or small continental

a few red cherry tomatoes to garnish
sea salt and black pepper

Blanch broccoli in boiling water for I minute, drain, rinse
Score cucumber skin with a fork, rinse under cold water and dice
Toss all ingredients together with no I dressing

tabouli with silver beet ♥

4 or more

I cup	burghal, cracked wheat
I cup	mint, chopped
I cup	parsley, chopped
I large	onion, finely chopped
4 small	young silver beet or spinach leaves
1/2 cup	lemon juice, fresh
1/2 cup	cold pressed olive oil
I cup	red cherry tomatoes (more if desired)

ground black pepper to taste

Soak burghal in 2 cups warm water for about 3/4 hour
Strain and pat dry on paper towelling
Soak silver beet leaves until they are crisp, trim stalks roughly chop
Mix burghal, mint, parsley, onion and silver beet together
Combine juice and oil and toss through salad
Add pepper to taste then add cherry tomatoes

mushroom plus salad ❤

serves 4 - 6

250g/9oz	button and field mushrooms, thinly sliced
1/2 cup	cashew, nuts chopped
1 small	red capsicum, seeded and thinly sliced
1 cup	mung bean sprouts
2 tbsp	garlic chives, chopped
1 dstsp	tamari

sea salt ground black pepper to taste.

Mix all ingredients together until combined
Gently toss in enough no 3 dressing until all ingredients are lightly coated

tomato salad ❤

4 or more

Great to eat as a snack with bread or serve with any mains hot or cold.

6	roma ripe tomatoes (long italian variety)
1 tbsp	basil leaves, chopped, fresh
1 small	onion, finely chopped
2 - 3 cloves	garlic, crushed
1 tsp	ground oregano
1/2 cup	lemon or lime juice, fresh

sea salt and ground black pepper to taste

Cut tomatoes
Sprinkle with oregano, stand for 15 minutes
Add all other ingredients
This combination gives tomatoes an exceptional flavour

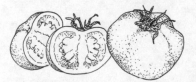

boiled egg salad & avocado dressing ❤

4 or more

6	hard boiled eggs, cut into quarters

paprika to garnish

dressing

1/2 cup	orange or apple juice
1/4 cup	lemon juice, fresh
1 large	avocado, peeled and stoned
1 clove	garlic, crushed
1 dstsp	mint, fresh

Mix dressing ingredients in a blender until smooth
Pour over eggs and sprinkle with paprika

simply carrots ❤

serves 2

Great on sandwiches, pocket pita bread and tacos
Will keep in a sealed container in the refrigerator for 1 or 2 days.

1 cup	carrots, grated or julienne sliced
1/2 cup	green beans, chopped or peas (cooked)
1 tbsp	water cress, chopped
1 tbsp	orange juice, fresh

grind some black pepper to your taste

Mix all ingredients together and serve

This salad is not only good for your liver, it will also improve your eyesight

coleslaw supreme ❤

serves 4 - 6

2 cups	cabbage, finely shredded (savoy or chinese)
1 cup	red cabbage, finely shredded
1 med	onion thinly sliced in half rings
1 small can	whole corn, drained
1 cup	carrot, grated or fine julienne strips
1 cup	pineapple, cut into small pieces, fresh or canned
1/2 cup	parsley roughly, chopped
1	lemon, juiced

sea salt and black pepper to taste

dressing

1/2 cup	natural soy yoghurt or soy mayonnaise
1/4 cup	orange juice, fresh
1/4 cup	light malt vinegar or lemon juice
1 tsp	chilli or hot English mustard (optional)

ground black pepper to taste

Blend all ingredients in dressing together, then toss through coleslaw
salad

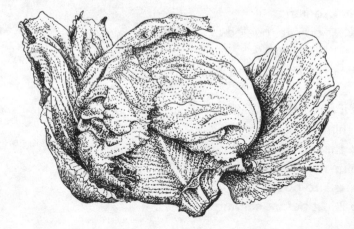

special potato salad ❤

4 or more

750g /27oz	new baby potatoes
1	red onion, thinly sliced in half rings
3 cloves	garlic, crushed
3	boiled eggs, chopped
3 tbsp	mint or coriander, fresh, chopped
2 tbsp	almonds, roasted, blanched, sliced

dressing
1/2 cup	natural soy yoghurt
1/2 cup	light malt vinegar or lemon juice
1 dstsp	honey, warmed for easy mixing
1 tsp	dijon mustard

sea salt and ground black pepper to taste

Mix dressing ingredients together until all combined
Wash potatoes, leave skin on and cut in half, cook until just tender
Gently mix all ingredients together then pour dressing over all

beaut beetroot salad ❤

4 or more

1 cup	beetroot, washed and trimmed
1 med	onion
1 large	orange, peeled of all pith
1/2 cup	pine nuts
1 clove	garlic, crushed

Beetroot is best if coarse grated or in very thin julienne strips
Slice onion into thin 1/2 rings
Slice orange into thin 1/2 slices
Slightly brown pine nuts in a non-stick pan
Toss all ingredients into bowl
Add dressing no 2 just before serving

Great with BBQ's, chicken or grilled fish

herb and spicy tomato bake ❤

4 or more

2 large	onions cut into very thin rings
820g/30oz	tomatoes, chopped (canned)
1 tbsp	basil, fresh, chopped
1 dstsp	cold pressed olive oil
2 cups	breadcrumbs (or ricecrumbs), fresh
1/2 tsp	mixed dried herbs
3 cloves	garlic, crushed
salt and ground black pepper to taste	

Separate onion rings and place in casserole dish
Mix basil with tomatoes, then place on top of onions
Rub oil into breadcrumbs and mixed herbs
Sprinkle breadcrumb mix on top of tomatoes
Bake casserole in a moderate oven for about 40 minutes until onion is tender and topping is golden brown

mashed potato with a difference ❤

4 or more

Ideal to serve with fish in place of chipped potatoes.

500g/18oz	potatoes, peeled, chopped and cooked in unsalted water until tender
1 dstsp	natural soy yoghurt
2	spring onions, finely chopped
2 tsp	horseradish
a little soy or oat milk	
sea salt and ground pepper to taste.	

Mash drained potato, yoghurt and enough milk to make a smooth mixture
Add onions, horseradish, salt and pepper

Can also be placed on top of a casserole. Rough the top of the potato with a fork and place under a griller until golden brown.

tasty potato bake ❤

serves 6 - 8

Ideal to serve with grilled or baked fish or a BBQ

1 kg/36oz	potatoes, peeled and thinly sliced
1 large	onion sliced in thin 1/2 rings
3 - 4 cloves	garlic, finely chopped
1 cup	chicken or vegetable stock
1 tbsp	natural soy yoghurt

sea salt and ground black pepper to taste
a little oil to brown garlic and onion

In an ovenproof dish arrange potato slices overlapping each other
Add browned onion and garlic, and black pepper to taste
Pour stock over potato
Cover casserole with foil, bake in moderate oven until potato is tender
Remove foil, spread yoghurt over potato, return to oven, brown
Add a little more water or stock if potato looks too dry

stuffed baked capsicums ❤

serves 4

2 large	red capsicums, cut into halves and deseeded
1 cup	rice, cooked
1 large	tomato, ripe, chopped
4 cloves	garlic, crushed
1/4 tsp	ground coriander
1/4 tsp	chilli powder (optional)
1 med	onion, finely chopped
1 tbsp	tamari

Place capsicum halves in an ovenproof dish
Mix all other ingredients together and spoon into capsicum halves
Cover dish with foil
Bake in a moderate oven for 1/2 hour or until vegetables are tender

bruschetta, summer tomatoes & basil

serves 6

This may seem obvious, but done traditionally it's to die for and will have you dreaming of tuscan villas on a hot summers day

10	vine ripened tomatoes
1 loaf	wood oven or crusty bread
3-4 cloves	garlic
10	basil leaves fresh (large)
1 + 1/2 tbsp	balsamic vinegar
cold pressed olive oil for blending	
sea salt and grindings of black pepper to taste	

Slice bread into wedges and brush on both sides with oil
Peel garlic and rub onto bread
Dice tomatoes
In a bowl, put vinegar, 2 tbsps olive oil, diced tomatoes and chopped basil leaves
Stir until mixture is well coated
Season with salt and pepper
Grill bread until golden brown on both sides
Place onto plates for serving
Spoon mixture onto bread and serve immediately

garlic, herb and chilli bread

2 whole	pita bread
1 whole	chilli, seeded and diced (optional)
3 - 4 cloves	garlic
2 tbsp	sesame seeds, toasted and crushed
1 tbsp	oregano, fresh or dried, diced
cold pressed olive oil for mixing	

Add all ingredients into a small bowl
Use a pastry brush to brush the mixture generously over one side of the bread
Bake in the oven until sizzling and serve immediately

vegetarian mains

stir fry beans with lemon and cashews

serves 2 - 4

This is a delicious dish when beans are in season and preferably when they are organic or home grown!

2 tbsp	cold pressed olive oil
handful	green beans, trimmed
handful	yellow beans, trimmed
handful	snowpeas, trimmed
2 cloves	garlic, finely sliced
3/4 cup	unsalted cashews
1 large	lemon, juiced
2 tbsp	palm sugar (optional)
2 tbsp	tamari
2 tbsp	mint (laksa) leaves
1 tbsp	ginger, grated
1 tbsp	lemongrass, finely chopped
2 cups	rice, cooked

Heat 2 tbsp olive oil in wok

Add garlic and cashews and stirfry for 1 minute

Add all beans and continue cooking for another two minutes or until crisp and tender

Add ginger, lemongrass, palm sugar, tamari and laksa mint and fry for another minute or two, until all ingredients are blended

Serve immediately on a bed of freshly steamed rice that has been cooked in vegetable stock, or water and a clove of garlic

tomato and fennel risotto

serves 2 - 4

Risotto is a meal in itself, for those craving a creamy textured meal. It is worth adding to your repertoire, although it may feel time consuming, when mastered you'll never look back!

6	roma tomatoes, slice lengthways, place on oven tray
440g/16oz	tomatoes (mashed), can
3 cups	vegetable stock
2 large	brown onions coarsely chopped
2 cloves	garlic, crushed
3 baby	fennel, sliced finely (around 1cm / 1/2 inch)
2 cups	italian aborio rice
1/2 tsp	rosemary dried

olive oil for stirfrying and roasting

Drizzle olive oil over tomatoes, sprinkle with rosemary, cracked pepper and some sea salt
Place in a moderate oven and roast until golden brown
In a heavy based saucepan, add two tablespoons of oil, and heat
When hot, add onions and garlic and stirfry for 2 minutes
Add the aborio rice and stirfry until clear, add the fennel and stir
Add tinned tomatoes and stir into mixture and allow to simmer
Put the stock into a jug and slowly add it to the mixture while stirring
Continue adding stock and stir until all the liquid is absorbed and the rice is soft and the risotto is creamy in texture (if you need more liquid use some extra vegetable stock)
Season with pepper and sea salt

Serve on a plate with the roasted roma tomatoes piled on top

lemon and basil pilaf with steamed asparagas

serves 2

To make this dish more substantial, serve with a green salad, a grilled chicken fillet basted in olive oil, or a fillet of fresh fish of your choice prepared in the same way!

2	onions finely chopped
2 cloves	garlic, crushed
1 tbsp	lemon rind, finely grated
2 cups	long grain rice
4+1/2 cups	vegetable stock
1/2 cup	basil leaves, chopped
1 bunch	fresh asparagus
cold pressed olive oil for cooking	

Use a deep frypan or heavy based saucepan and heat two tbsps oil
Add garlic and onions and cook until golden
Add lemon rind and rice to pan and cook until rice is translucent
Pour in the stock and basil, simmer for 15 minutes or until stock is absorbed and rice is soft
To prepare the asparagus, place washed bunch in steamer on stove for 3 minutes when water begins to boil
You can toss asparagus in olive oil, lemon juice and tamari before serving

Serve pilaf on plate topped with asparagus, and a green salad.
Season to taste and enjoy.

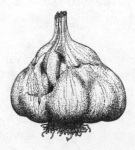

susan's summer pasta

serves 4

1/2 cup	cold pressed olive oil
500g / 18oz	tomatoes, firm and ripe, finely chopped
2 small	onions, finely chopped
10	green olives, pitted and chopped
4	black olives, pitted and chopped
2 cloves	garlic, crushed
1/3 cup	parsley chopped
1 tbsp	capers
1/4 tsp	oregano, fresh
2 tbsp	sesame seeds, toasted
1 packet	pasta, big shells to catch the sauce

Cook the pasta
Combine all ingredients into a bowl
Mix well, allow mixture to stand over night, in the refrigerator
Sprinkle with toasted sesame seeds, serve cold mixture over warm pasta

basic tomato pasta sauce

serves 4

2 cups	chopped tomatoes, or a can
1	onion, thinly sliced
2 cloves	garlic
1 tbsp	tomato paste
1 cup	vegetable stock or water
1 cup	parsley, chopped
black pepper and sea salt to taste	

Heat fry pan, add tomato paste and stir for 1 - 2 minutes
Add oil, onion, garlic and cook for approx 5 minutes
Add tomatoes, and water or stock, cook for 10 miutes
Just before serving, add the parsley, stir in for 30 seconds
A basic sauce, experiment with other flavours, ie. chilli, bay leaves

tomato tart

serves 6

You will need a pastry base for this recipe, (see page 263 or 276)
Great for picnics, parties and lunches

4 tbsp	cold pressed olive oil
I clove	garlic,crushed
450g/16oz	tomatoes, ripe
I	egg, just yolk beaten
handful	basil leaves, sliced into strips
I can	anchovies, flat (optional)
black pepper and salt to taste	

Preheat the oven to 200°C/390°F
Combine olive oil and garlic in a small bowl, set aside
Core, slice and seed tomatoes, drain on kitchen paper
Arrange pastry on a baking sheet
Put pastry onto a pie dish, push into the corners
Bake the dough for 10 mins, until slightly golden
Brush the pastry with the garlic oil mixutre
Sprinkle with half the basil
Season with black pepper and salt
Arrange the tomatoes, in the pie dish
Pour the remaining garlic oil mixture over the tomatoes
Arrange the anchovies in a decorative circle
Bake for a further 10-15 mins, until the tomatoes are soft
Allow to cool

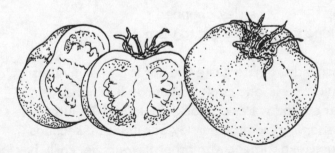

hero vegetable stew

serves 4

1 bunch	asparagus, trimmed and cut into lengths
8 small	zucchini, ends trimmed
12 baby	carrots, trimmed and peeled
8	pearl onions, peeled
1 cup	peas, fresh from the pod
6 baby	turnips, peeled and topped
1	shallot, peeled and finley chopped
700ml/24oz	vegetable stock
2 med	tomatoes
2 tbsp	cold pressed olive oil
15	basil leaves
salt and black pepper to taste	

Blanch the asparagus, zucchini, carrots, peas, turnips and pearl onions
separately in salted water
Don't over cook them, they must be quite crisp
Drain and run under cold water
In a large pan, sauté the shallots in 2 tbsp of oil
Add stock and bring to the boil
Simmer to reduce the quantity of water by at least half
Add diced tomatoes
Simmer for 3 minutes
Add the remaining vegetables and heat for a further 4 minutes
Season with salt and pepper
Sprinkle with the basil and serve in shallow bowls

Serve with crusty or toasted turkish bread and a big green salad

AUDREY TEA HINT
Be confident when you cook!

chunky roast vegetables ♥

serves 4

This dish is also great cold!

2 large	peppers, yellow and red, seeded, cut into thick strips
4 small	eggplants, trimmed, cut lengthways into quarters
6 small	potatoes, depending on how small, cut into quarters
3 med	onions, peeled and cut into quarters
2 bunches	asparagus, ends cut
10 cloves	garlic, whole, peeled
6 sprigs	thyme
4 sprigs	rosemary
3 tbsp	olive oil

salt and ground black pepper

Preheat the oven to its highest setting
Put all the vegetables into two trays
Toss in the garlic and herbs, over the two trays
Season with salt and pepper
Drizzle the oil over the vegetables, lightly
Bake for approx 20 - 30 minutes in a moderate oven

Serve alone, or with the tomato tart, big salad or fish.

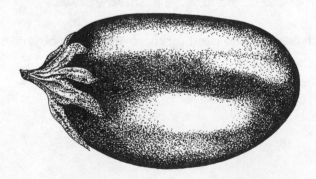

pumpkin couscous

serves 4

150g/5-6oz	couscous
200ml/7oz	water
1/2 tsp	saffron threads
250ml/8-9oz	vegetable stock
4 tbsp	cold pressed olive oil
1 med	onion
400g/14oz	pumpkin, very orange, diced
1 large	lemon, juice, keep the rind, thinly slice
1 stick	cinnamon
2	bay leaves
2 tbsp	LSA, coursley ground
4 sprigs	mint

salt and black pepper to taste

Put the couscous into a mixing bowl.
Boil the water and pour over the couscous and leave for 15 mins
Add the saffron to the stock and set aside
Heat 3 tbsp of the oil in a saucepan
Add the onion and fry until almost clear
Add pumpkin, stirfry for 2 minutes
Drain the couscous and add to the pan with the saffron liquid
Add lemon rind, cinnamon, bay leaves and salt and pepper
Bring to the boil, then simmer, reduce the liquid until nearly evaporated
Remove the cinnamon, bay leaves and lemon rind
Mix in the LSA

Serve with the mint leaves on top

lentil and vegetable loaf ♥

serves 4

440g/16oz	kidney beans, canned, drained, rinsed
2 cups	mashed potato
2	zucchini, grated
1	carrot, grated
1	onion, grated
1 tbsp	LSA
1 tbsp	natural soy yoghurt
1	egg, beaten
1/2 cup	bread crumbs (can be wheat free)

salt and ground black pepper to taste

dressing

1/2 cup	natural soy yoghurt
1 tbsp	chives, fresh chopped.

Mash beans with a fork in a large bowl
Stir in all other ingredients and mix well
Press mixture into oiled loaf tin
Top with breadcrumbs and bake for 25/30 minutes, in a moderate oven.
Cut into slices and serve topped with dressing

Serve with steamed carrots, zucchini, snow peas and a big green salad.

Not suitable for freezing

stroganoff without meat ❤

serves 4

440g/16oz	lima beans, canned, drained, rinsed,
1 tbsp	garlic, crushed
440g/16oz	tomatoes, canned
1 med	onion, chopped
2 med	zucchini, grated
1 cup	broccoli, chopped
1 med	capsicum, seeded, cut into thin strips
2 tbsp	tomato paste
1/2 cup	vegetable stock
400g/14oz	button or field mushrooms, washed
1 cup	soy yoghurt
1	bay leaf

sea salt and cracked pepper to taste

Combine all ingredients except mushrooms and yoghurt.
Place in a covered casserole dish
Bake in a moderate oven for 45 minutes.
Add mushrooms, cook further 15 minutes
Before serving stir in soy yoghurt.

Serve with crusty bread and a big green salad

Be confident and fearless as a cook. Accept compliments and criticisms graciously.
Never apologise, just do your best. Audrey Tea

spicy pasta ❤

serves 4

250g/9oz	dry wholemeal spiral pasta
1 large	carrot, cut into thin strips
1 stick	celery, cut into thin strips
1	red capsicum, cut into thin strips
1/2 cup	broccoli, chopped
1/2	green beans, chopped
4 small	chillies, whole stems on
1/4 cup	no 2 dressing (page 192)
1 tsp	curry paste of your choice
2 tsp	tumeric powder

Add pasta to boiling water and boil uncovered until pasta is just tender, drain. Steam vegetables until crispy tender, drain
Mix dressing & spices together and gently toss through pasta and vegetables.
Serve with a big green salad and crusty bread

broad beans ❤

serves 4

If you have never enjoyed broad beans before, give this a try because these beans are delicious and have many health benefits

500g /18oz	broad beans - fresh or frozen
440g/16oz	tomatoes, canned
3 cloves	garlic, crushed (optional)
2 tbsp	basil , fresh chopped (mint if you do not like basil)
1 large	onion, chopped

Ground black pepper and sea salt to taste

Cook beans until tender then drain
Brown onion and garlic in pan with a little cold pressed olive oil
Add beans and tomato to pan, add basil and simmer for 5 minutes
Season to taste

tangy tasty lunch mexican style ♥

serves 4 - 6

450g/16oz	kidney beans, canned, drained
1 large	onion, chopped
3 large	cloves garlic, chopped
1 tbsp	cold pressed olive oil
1 tbsp	tomato paste (more if desired)
1 tsp	oregano, fresh
1 tbsp	parsley, chopped
1 tbsp	basil, chopped
1 pinch	chilli powder and paprika (optional)
a little water	
sea salt and cracked pepper to taste	

Brown onion and garlic in oil in large pan
Add all other ingredients plus enough water to bind together
Don't make it too moist, warm through
Serve with taco shells, burritos or nachos, chopped tomatoes, sliced
lettuce, alfalfa sprouts and chilled soy yoghurt

basic vegetable stock

5 cups	water
5	black peppercorns
1	onion, skin on and cut in half
2	carrot, whole
2	tomato, washed and halved
2	bay leaves
2 stalks	celery
1 tsp	sea salt
2 tbsp	cold pressed olive oil

In a hot heavy saucepan, add oil
When hot add all ingredients except water
Keep ingredients moving so they don't stick and burn, for 5 minutes
Add water, bring to the boil, then simmer for an hour. Strain
Use immediately or cool, then refrigerate

zucchini slice ❤

serves 4

This slice can also be cut into wedges and served cold for a picnic as finger food.

5 large	eggs, lightly beaten
400g/14oz	zucchini, coarsely grated
2 med	carrots, coarsely grated
1 large	onion, finely chopped
2 cloves	garlic, crushed (optional)
1/2 cup	cold pressed olive oil
1/2 cup	parsley, chopped
1/2 tsp	lemon juice
1 cup	wholemeal SR flour
100g/4oz	soft tofu
1 tbsp	LSA

salt and ground black pepper to taste

Combine all ingredients except the flour until well mixed
Fold in flour until well blended.
Pour into an oiled lamington tin 28 x 18cm (12"x 8")
Bake in a moderate oven for 30 to 40 minutes.
Serve warm with a fresh salad and rice.

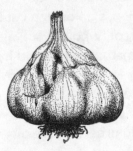

AUDREY TEA HINT
All frozen serves should be placed in the freezer as soon as possible.
This is a very practical and economical way to save on cooking time and yet
have a quickly prepared tasty meal.

almost a nori roll

makes approx 10 rolls

You will need a sushi mat for this recipe, which you can get from some supermarkets or an Asian grocery store. Try using different ingredients like prawns, tofu, tuna. Great for lunches, entrees, snacks

5 sheets	nori seaweed
1 med	avocado
1 bunch	garlic chives
2	lebanese cucumbers
5 tbsp	LSA
2 tbsp	sesame seeds, dry roasted
1 tube	wasabi (horseradish paste)
1 pkt	pickled ginger (optional)
4 tbsp	tamari
5 cups	brown or basmati rice, cooked

While the rice is still warm stir through the LSA and sesame seeds
Let the rice sit while you prepare the other ingredients
Peel the avocado and slice into strips
Wash and separate the garlic chives
Cut the cucumber into long thin strips
Put the nori sheet on the sushi mat
Cover the nori with a thin layer of rice -
Leave about 2cm (3/4 inch) clear at the top and bottom of the nori.
Fill to the sides
Spread a thin strip of wasabi along the centre of the rice
At the end closest to you place 3 strips of garlic chives
Put a strip of cucumber next then a strip of avocado
Roll the mat up, away from you, creating a compact roll
Be careful not to roll the mat into the nori roll
You can cut the long rolls into bite size pieces or just in half
Use a wet knife to do so

Serve with pickled ginger, a dipping sauce of wasabi stirred into the tamari and a big green salad

tofu and tempeh salad ❤

serves 4

390g/14oz	tempeh
340g/12oz	tofu
1 cup	bean sprouts
1	green chilli
3	spring onions
2 tsp	ginger root, grated
2	garlic cloves, crushed
1 tbsp	mild vinegar or lemon juice
1 tbsp	tamari
1/2 tsp	mustard, hot (optional)
6 tbsp	water
4 tbsp	cold pressed olive oil

ground black pepper and salt to taste

Cut the tofu and tempeh into thin strips.
Wash the bean sprouts
Heat the oil and stir fry the tofu and tempeh until golden brown.
Set the tofu and tempeh aside
In the same pan, stir fry the spring onions, chillies, ginger and garlic for about 1 minute
Add the water and bring to the boil
Turn the heat down and simmer for 2 minutes
Add the tofu and tempeh, stir and add the bean sprouts
Simmer for a further 2 minutes

Serve hot or cold on a bed of rice with a big salad

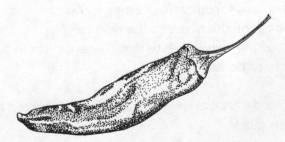

vegetable and tofu quiche

serves 4

Great cold for a lunchbox
Have a partially cooked pie crust ready (pages 263 or 276)

2 tbsp	cold pressed olive oil
2 tsp	garlic, crushed, optional
1 tbsp	ginger root minced
2 cups	shallots chopped
1 cup	fennel chopped
1 cup	broccoli chopped
1/2 cup	carrots diced
600 g/22oz	tofu - firm
1	egg
4 tbsp	parsley, basil finely diced

Salt and ground black pepper to taste

Heat the oil in a frypan add garlic, ginger and shallots
Cook until the shallots are transparent
Add the fennel, broccoli and carrots
Cook until soft. If the vegies start to stick add a little bit of water
Drop the tofu into some boiling water for 1 minute, drain well
Blend the tofu with egg, salt and herbs to form a smooth cream
Combine all the vegies and tofu mixture
Pour into the ready pie crust
Bake for approx 30 mins (180°C/350°F) or until the quiche has risen
and set. Could take a little longer

warm green salad

serves 2

2 bunches	asparagus
2 cups	sugar snap peas, stringed
3 tbsp	cold pressed olive oil
2 tbsp	lemon juice
2 cups	broccoli, large florets
2 cups	snow peas, stringed
6 baby	potatoes, washed, steamed and cut into quarters

ground black pepper and sea salt to taste

Place cooked potatoes in the big salad bowl
Prepare the other vegetables. String the peas
Do not take the peas from the shell. Keep them whole
Discard the ends of the asparagus
Place all the green vegies into the steamer
When the broccoli goes bright green, turn off the heat
Put the green vegies on top of the potatoes
Drizzle the olive oil and lemon juice over the top

Can be served on a bed or rice, couscous or amaranth
Delicious by itself with some or your favourite bread

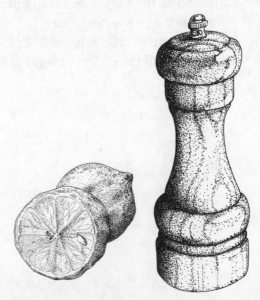

baked polenta

serves 4 or more

Polenta can be firm or soft like mash potato. It is a very versitile food like pasta or bread.

1 large	onion, chopped
3 cups	stock, chicken or vegetable
3 tbsp	cold pressed olive oil
2 cloves	garlic, crushed
1 cup	polenta, finely ground (maybe more)
1 cup	rice milk (or water)
ground black pepper and salt to taste	

Heat the saucepan and pour in the oil
Add the onion and garlic, on a medium heat, till clear
Then pour all the liquid into the pan
Turn up to high till liquid simmers
Slowly add the polenta in a thin stream
Stir constantly
When all the polenta is added, turn the heat down to very low
If it is too high the polenta will spit and pop
Cover with a lid and cook on very low for another 10-15 minutes
When the polenta is cooked spoon into a rectangular cake tin
It will set into a firm loaf that can be cut

It can be cut into thick slices and served immediately with any pasta sauce or taken to work for lunch. It reheats extremely well in the microwave

For variation, it is lovely warm with a big salad, and/or tuna or sardines with lemon juice and tamari dressing

If you don't want it to be firm then do not use as much polenta. Experiment and see what consistancy you prefer.

Keep leftovers in the refrigerator

poultry

stir fry chicken with lime leaves

serves 4

A tasty stir fry with the clean fresh taste of kaffir lime leaves

2 tbsp	sesame oil
6	shallots, finely chopped
1 tbsp	freshly grated ginger
8	lime leaves (try kaffir lime leaves), finely shredded
4	chicken fillets, sliced into thin strips
3 tbsp	tamari
1 tbsp	red miso
2 bunches	bok choy (asian, green leafy vegetable)
4 tbsp	basil, (thai is best for this resipe) torn
2 cups	rice, cooked

In a wok, heat sesame oil and add shallots, ginger, lime leaves and chicken
Add the tamari, miso and bok choy and stir through
Keep the wok moving over heat, cook until the chicken is tender
Stir through basil and serve on a bed of steamed rice
(try cooking the rice with coconut milk instead of water for an authentic
Asian flavour!)

Serve with a green salad

COOKING HINT FOR STIRFRY:
The secret to a good stirfry is to heat the wok first, add the oil or stock (if
you would rather avoid the oil). Add the ingredients immediately to the oil,
so that the oil does not get burnt. Keep the heat high and the food moving
in the wok.

summer chicken kebabs

serves 4

Something for the BBQ or under the grill on balmy summer nights

marinade

1/3 cup	cold pressed olive oil
2	spring onions, finely chopped
1	chilli, fresh finely sliced
2 tbsp	coriander, chopped
1 tsp	ground tumeric
1 tsp	ground cumin
2 tbsp	tamari
1 tsp	palm sugar (optional)
1 tbsp	lime or lemon juice
4	chicken breast fillets, cut into bite sized pieces
24	button mushrooms

stainless steel or wooden skewers from supermarket

Combine all marinade ingredients into a large bowl and stir well
Add chicken pieces to marinade, cover and refrigerate for 2 hours
When ready to cook, take a skewer and thread chicken and mushrooms
alternately until all 8 skewers are prepared
Barbecue, or grill, turning occasionally for 8 mins or until chicken is tender

Serve with your favourite summer salad
Alternatively you could replace the chicken with fish or tofu!

chicken omelette and rice

serves 2

4 large	free range eggs
1 med	zuchini, grated
2 cups	basmati rice (cooked)
1 cup	chicken fillets, cut into thin strips
2 tbsp	fish sauce
2 tsp	sambal (chillis in vinegar), or fresh chilli (optional)
1 cup	chicken stock
1	spring onion tops, chopped.

peanut or cold pressed olive oil for frying

Use a frypan or wok
Put half oil heat and quickly cook the chicken
Remove the chicken from the pan
Crack the eggs and put into a mixing bowl
Put the zucchini, chicken and fish sauce into the bowl
Whisk or beat the ingredients
In the wok place 1 tbsp oil, heat and swirl around
Place half the ingredients and swirl around, flip over when brown
Repeat for the other side
Do exactly the same for the other omelette
Heat the chicken stock

Serve on a mound of rice, place the omelette next to it
Add 1 teaspoon of sambal (optional but delicious)
In 2 small bowls pour the chicken stock and sprinkle with spring onions
The stock is delicious poured onto the rice

Serve with a large side salad

grilled chicken and fig salad

serves 2-4

A dish to enjoy for lunch or dinner

2 large	chicken breasts
1	eggplant sliced in 1cm(1/2 inch) rounds
8	raddichio leaves (a bitter yet tasty lettuce style plant, with purple blush to the leaves)
6	fresh figs, halved
	cold pressed olive oil for cooking

dressing
lemon juice, honey, marjoram leaves
pepper and sea salt if required

In a jar, squeeze the juice of one medium lemon,
1 tbsp of honey, 1\2 cup of marjoram leaves, a dash of tamari, sea salt and pepper to taste
(if you like garlic, crush one clove into the mixture)

Put a lid on the jar and shake until blended and set aside
Baste the chicken fillets and eggplant in olive oil and grill until chicken is tender and eggplant is golden brown (the chicken may need to go under the grill first)
Wash and pat dry raddichio leaves
Arrange two leaves on each of 4 plates
When chicken and eggplant is cooked, slice chicken into long thickish strips
Pile chicken and eggplant onto leaves and top with fresh figs
Shake dressing and pour onto salad

For best results serve while still warm

poached chicken breasts with spring vegetables

serves 4

300ml/10oz	chicken stock
2 cloves	garlic, finely chopped
4	chicken breasts
1 tbsp	basil pesto
1 bunch	water cress, washed and set aside
1 tbsp	chives chopped
100 g/4oz	baby carrots, washed
100 g/4oz	shelled broad beans
6	baby zucchini, topped tailed, sliced lengthways

salt and pepper to taste

Put chicken stock, water cress, pesto,some salt and pepper into a food processor
Blend until smooth
In a large saucepan place the zucchini, baby carrots and broad beans
Sprinkle with garlic and chives
Lay the chicken on top of the vegetables
Pour the sauce over the top and cover
Simmer for 30 to 40 mins or until chicken is tender

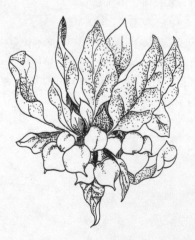

chicken and vegetable stirfry

serves 4 - 6

A meal in itself. The dried mushrooms are necessary for the flavour.
Quantities of vegetables can be added or taken out as desired
A nourishing and cleansing meal

1 tbsp	cold pressed olive oil
2 tbsp	tamari
1200 ml/40oz	chicken stock
6 to 8	shiitake mushrooms, soaked in warm water, 30 mins or field/button mushrooms
3	chicken fillets, sliced finely
8 fresh	asparagus spears, chopped into 2.5cm (1inch)pieces
12	green beans, chopped into 2.5cm (1 inch) pieces
14	sugar snap peas, washed
1 handful	bean and/or snowpea sprouts
125g/4-5oz	noodles, yellow asian noodles, boiled for 2 minutes

Warm the stock in a large saucepan while you cook the stirfry
Just before you begin cooking, put the cooked noodles into the warming stock to heat before serving
Heat the oil in a wok or deep frypan
Add asparagus and beans and stirfry for 2 mins
Add chicken and fry for another 2 mins
Drain mushrooms, add to stirfry along with peas
Stir for another two mins
Stir through tamari and bean sprouts and turn off heat
Place equal portions stock and noodles into large soup bowls
Put spoonfuls of stir fry into the bowls

warm chicken salad with turkish bread

serves 3 - 4

Positively lip smacking!

4 tbsp	cold pressed olive oil
2	cloves garlic crushed
500g/18oz	cherry tomatoes, washed
4	lebanese cucumbers. cut thinly lengthways
200g/7oz	artichokes, tinned, drained and quartered
100g/3-4oz	caperberries, drained (small)
3	chicken breast fillets, poached and sliced
2 tbsp	basil leaves, chopped
3 tbsp	cider vinegar or lemon
1 to 2	loaves turkish bread, cut into large triangles

to poach chicken
In a non-stick frypan put 4 tablespoons of chicken stock or water
with a bay leaf
Bring to boil
Place the chicken breasts and turn down to a gentle simmer until
cooked

Combine tomato, cucumber, chicken, caperberries, artichokes and herbs
into a large bowl
Combine olive oil, cider vinegar, and garlic and pour over salad
Gently mix salad and set aside
Brush bread with olive oil and grill on both sides until golden brown
Put spoonfuls of salad onto bread and serve on large platter or individual
plates

Season with salt and pepper to taste

celebration chicken, stuffed and boned

serves 4 - 6

Order the boned chicken from your butcher 3- 4 days prior
This dish can be cooked one day in advance or hours beforehand
Delicious cold for picnics and sliced for sandwiches and parties

6 tbsp	cold pressed olive oil
1	chicken young roasting (1.1kg/40oz) boned,

stuffing

6 slices	bread, cut into bite size pieces
8 tbsp	milk (soy, oat or rice)
450g/16oz	chicken minced
1 bunch	parsley, fresh finely chopped
2 cloves	garlic, finely chopped
salt and pepper to taste	

a large darning needle, some strong cotton thread, doubled over
Ask your butcher to mince the chicken, from fresh fillets, while you are in the shop.

Preheat oven to 180°C/350°F
Put the diced bread and milk into a bowl, soak for 10 to 15 minutes
Put the minced chicken, chopped garlic, parsley and pepper into a large bowl, mix thoroughly
Combine both mixtures, mix thoroughly with your hands
Lay the boned chicken skin side down on a clean work surface
Stuff the leg cavities, mould them to look like chicken legs
Stuff the body cavity, stitch as you go, so the stuffing doesn't fall out
Overlap the flesh and skin so the stitches do not tear open
Continue until all stuffing is used and the chicken is securely stitched
Use a generous, deep sided baking dish with 3 - 6 tbsps olive oil
Place the bird, stitched side down, cook for 30 mins
Gently turn bird, be careful not to tear skin, brown the other side
Partially cover bird with a lid so as to not burn (baste occasionally)
Once chicken is cooked (1 + 1/2 hours), remove from oven, rest for 10 minutes before serving

Serve already carved, so that guests can see the stuffing

chicken meatloaf

serves 6

Use all of the ingredients for the stuffing from the "celebration chicken" recipe. Use the same quantities. See page 237.

Grease a terrine dish or log tin in olive oil
Place all mixture into tin
Cover with foil and bake in 180°C/350°F oven for 3\4 to 1 hour
Delicious and filling this meatloaf can be used as a meal served with a big green salad. Also great for picnics and sandwich fillings

lemon and herb chicken marinade

serves 4

4 pieces	chicken (maryland cut)
1/2 cup	cold pressed olive oil
1 + 1/2	lemons juiced
2 cloves	garlic, crushed
2 tsp	french tarragon, dried
2 tsp	basil, dried
sprigs of the above herbs for edible decoration	

Marinade chicken in oil, lemon juice and garlic for 2 hours in the refrigerator
Pre heat oven 180°C/350°F
Bake chicken in the marinade with the herbs, basting occasionally
Cook for 10 to 15 mins or until chicken is tender
You can also cook on a BBQ for a delicious summer treat

Serve with your best green salad!

singapore noodles

serves 4 - 6

3 tbsp	olive oil
3 cloves	garlic ,crushed
2	red chillis, finely chopped (optional)
3	spring onions, finely chopped
250ml/8oz	fish stock
250g/9oz	chicken, cooked thinly sliced
300g/11oz	small prawns
2 tsp	salted soy bean paste, mixed with 1 tbsp water, or 3 tsp soy sauce without adding extra water
2 cups	white chinese cabbage, sliced finely cross ways
500g/18oz	hokkien mee noodles
250g/9oz	bean sprouts
1 handful	baby spinach leaves
2 tbsp	tamari

Heat oil in wok or large pan and stirfry garlic until golden
Remove garlic from pan with slotted spoon and set aside for garnish
Stirfry the chillis in the oil then add prawns and soybean paste
Stirffy for 2 minutes then add cabbage and spring onions
Add fish stock, noodles, bean sprouts and spinach leaves
Continue to cook and simmer for 2 minutes, turning slowly
Stir through tamari and put into individual bowls
Garnish with garlic and cucumber for a rewarding flavour combination!

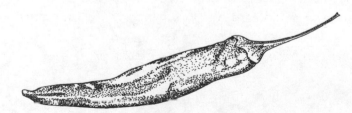

thai green chicken curry

serves 4

350g/12-13oz	chicken, chopped into pieces
1 tbsp	thai green curry paste (you might like more)
1 tbsps	cold pressed olive oil
1 cup	green peas (fresh)
1 cup	green beans, tipped and left whole
1 cup	coconut cream
1/2 cup	coriander
1 tbsp	lemon, chopped very finely
2 whole	red chillis (optional)
2 cups	rice, cooked

Heat oil in a non-stick pan on medium-low heat
Add curry paste and heat for one minute
Add half the coconut milk and cook until oil appears on the top
Add chicken pieces and cook for around 10 minutes or until done
Add the remaining coconut milk, green peas, beans and lemons
Simmer until tender
Garnish with sprigs of coriander

Serve with boiled rice and fresh garden salad

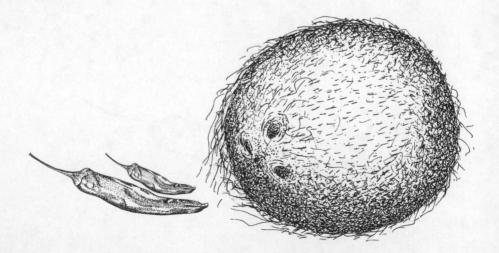

apricot fat free chicken ♥

serves 4

4 large	chicken breast fillets, trimmed of all fat
4 tbsp	dried apricots, chopped
2 tbsp	hazelnuts, chopped
I tsp	dried oregano (if fresh, triple the amount, dice)
2 cloves	garlic, chopped
Sea salt and freshly ground black pepper	

Mix apricots, nuts and oregano
Cut the chicken fillets to open out as flat as possible
Lay one fillet out and sprinkle 1/4 of filling over the flesh, repeat for the other 3 fillets
Sprinkle top fillet with ground black pepper and a little oregano
Tie fillets into a parcel shape with string and place into oven bag
Add 2 tablespoons of apricot nectar or water to oven bag
Bake in oven as directed - about I hour or until tender
After cooking, snip bag and retain juices, make juices up to I cup with water, and use as a tasty sauce
Slice your chicken parcel carefully with a sharp knife

basic chicken stock

500g/18oz	chicken, wings, bones, legs (free range)
5 cups	water
5	black peppercorns
I	onion, skin on and cut in half
I	carrot, whole
2 stalks	celery
I tsp	sea salt
2 tbsp	cold pressed olive oil

In a hot heavy saucepan, add oil
When hot add all ingredients except water
Keep ingredients moving so they don't stick and burn, for about 5 minutes
Add water, bring to the boil, then simmer for an hour. Strain
Let cool and scrape off the fat, refrigerate or reheat to use

seafood

scallops with grape fruit juice

serves 4

2 cloves	garlic, crushed
I cup	grapefruit juiced
4	spring onions, finely sliced
I tsp	cold pressed walnut oil (or olive oil)
48	scallops on I\2 shell

Combine garlic, grapefruit juice, onion and oil
Place scallops in shells in a single layer on an oven tray
Spoon some of the mixture over scallops
Add freshly ground pepper and grill for 5 mins
Toss in a bowl with remaining juice and devour
Serve with a tossed salad and steamed potatoes

grilled korma curry and spiced snapper

serves 4

2 whole	baby snapper, cleaned & gutted
1/3 cup	Korma Curry Paste
1/2 cup	slithered almonds
1/2 cup	coriander leaves, chopped finely
I	lime, cut into wedges for garnish
I tbsp	cold pressed olive oil

Slice each snapper on both sides 3-4 times diagonally
Preheat grill or barbecue
In a small bowl combine together the Korma curry paste, slithered almonds and coriander, baste over fish
Grill snapper on both sides until centre is cooked
Brush citrus pieces with oil and lightly grill- serve with snapper

Serve with rice and salad

tuna and potato salad

serves 2 or more

1/4 cup	cold pressed olive oil
2 tbsp	tamari (wheat free soy sauce)
1	red salad onion, peeled and sliced finely
225g/8oz	tuna good quality
1/2	iceburg lettuce, washed and torn up
1 clove	garlic, crushed
1	lemon juiced
1	lebanese cucumber, sliced lengthways
1 punnet	cherry tomatoes, washed
8 small	tomatoes, chopppped
4	eggs, hard boiled and quartered
8 small	new potatoes, steamed, left to cool, then quartered

Combine oil, tamari, lemon juice and some salt and set aside
Put remaining ingredients into a large serving bowl and mix gently
Pour dressing over salad and set aside for 5 mins before serving

Serve this delicious and nutritious meal with your favourite crusty bread!

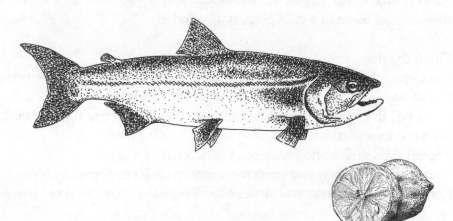

tuna and rice hotpot

serves 4

4	tuna steaks
1 + 1/2 cups	basmati rice
1/2 tsp	sea or celtic salt
3 tbsp	cold pressed olive oil
1/2 tsp	chilli powder (optional)
1 tbsp	lemon juice
2	onions finely chopped
450g/16oz	button mushrooms sliced
2 tbsp	ginger root grated
2 large	tomatoes skinned & chopped
450g/16oz	spinach washed/shredded
2 - 4 large	red chillis seeded (optional)
2 cups	fish stock or water

Ground black pepper and sea salt to taste

Soak the rice in cold water for 2 hours (makes it soft)
Rub the tuna with salt, chilli powder and lemon juice
Put the steaks on a plate in the fridge

To make salsa -
Stirfry onions in the oil until soft. Add mushrooms, cook for 1 minute.
Add chillis (if used), ginger, tomatoes and seasoning, cook for another 5 minutes. Set aside in a cool place until needed

Drain the rice.
In a large pot with a tight fitting lid put the stock or water and rice, bring to the boil. Turn the heat down, simmer for 10 minutes
Place half the spinach on top of the rice, then half of the tomato salsa, then the tuna steaks
Repeat the spinach and finally the tomato salsa on top
Cover the top tightly and cook for another 15-20 minutes
Remove from the heat and let it sit for 5 minutes on a damp tea towel

Serve with a big green salad.

tuna and basil gnocchi

serves 3

1/2 bunch	basil washed and torn
250g/8oz	tuna and oil
3 tbsp	lemon juice
500g/18oz	gnocchi (little balls of potato and/or wheat)
ground black pepper and sea salt to taste	

In a big salad bowl put the lemon juice, basil and tuna
Bring to the boil 2 litres/70oz of water
Put the gnocchi in when the water is boiling
When the gnocchi floats to the top, wait 1 minute and scoop out
Place in the bowl with the other ingredients
Mix well. Be careful not to crush the gnocchi
(Gnocchi can be bought from a supermarket or homemade)

tuna salad

serves 4

A meal for eating from a big bowl all on your own

250g/8oz	tuna in brine (good)
1 handful	black olives, pitted
8 large	lettuce leaves, washed and torn up
1	spring onion finely sliced
2	hard boiled eggs, halved
3	ripe tomatoes diced

dressing

1 tbsp	olive oil
1 tbsp	tamari
1/2	lemon, juiced

In a large bowl combine all ingredients, except the eggs
Shake dressing and pour over salad
Add eggs and season to taste. Simple as that!

marinated tuna with grapefruit, noodles and asparagus

serves 4 - 6

2	grapefruit, peeled and segmented
I	grapefruit juiced
I tbsp	cider vinegar (lemon juice)
I clove	garlic, crushed
1/2 cup	sesame oil, cold pressed
1/4 cup	walnut oil or cold pressed olive oil
4	spring onions, finely sliced
	(chill in cold water to curl onion, drain, set aside)
I kg/36oz	tuna steak, slice across the grain, as fine as possible
	(try partially freezing the tuna to make slicing easier)
I tsp	cold pressed olive oil
I bunch	aspargus spears, trimmed and halved
	(blanched in boiling water and set aside)
250g/9oz	cellophane noodles or rice noodles

Combine grapefruit juice, cider vinegar, garlic, walnut, sesame oil, and half the spring onions into a bowl

Place the tuna in a shallow ceramic dish, pour over half the marinade (refrigerate for 2 hours or longer, turn the tuna at least once)

Cook noodles in a large saucepan of boiling water for 5 mins

Drain and rinse under cold water

Toss noodles in olive oil

In a non-stick fry pan, very quickly sear the tuna on both sides

Pile the noodles onto a plate and place tuna on top

Place the grapefruit, asparagus and remaining green onions onto the tuna

Spoon on remaining marinade

Serve on a large platter as part of a banquet or with a big vegetable salad

fresh fish with ginger and spring onions

serves 4

Tuna, atlantic salmon or salmon trout are the preferred choices for this refreshing meal.
Try wrapping the fish in fresh banana leaves instead of foil. Available at Asain green grocers and in some supermarkets.

4 pieces	fish of your choice, fresh
4 tsp	cold pressed olive oil
3	spring onions, sliced cross ways
I small piece	ginger, freshly grated
4 pieces	foil or banana leaves for wrapping fish
thinly sliced lemon wedges for garnish	

Preheat oven to 180°C/350°F
Place a piece of fish onto the foil or leaf
Spoon over 1 tsp oil, some ginger, spring onions and a lemon wedge
Loosely cover with foil or wrap in banana leaves
Repeat the process 3 more times for other pieces of fish
Place all parcels in an oven proof dish
Bake for 15 to 20 mins
When ready season with salt and pepper to taste

Serve with a fresh cucumber salad

Getting together is a beginning. Keeping together is progress.
Working together is success. Henry Ford

marinated calamari ❤

serves 4

This dish is best made the day before you need it

500g/18oz	calamari, small tubes are more tender!
1/3 cup	cold pressed olive oil
1 clove	garlic, finely chopped
1/3 cup	lemon juice
2 tbsp	parsley, chopped

Wash squid under cold running water and pat dry
Slice into 1cm (1/2 inch) rings
Bring a large saucepan of water to the boil and drop in the squid
Reduce the heat and simmer for 5 minutes, drain and set aside
In a bowl, combine oil, lemon juice and squid,
Cover and refrigerate over night
When ready to serve, add the garlic and parsley to the marinade
Mix well and let stand for two hours, season to taste

Serve in the marinade at the table with a big green salad!

basic fish stock

2 kg/4.4lbs	fish bones, heads (white fish), rinsed
2 tbsp	cold pressed olive oil
1	carrot
2 stalks	celery
10	black peppercorns
1 strip	lemon peel
5 cups	water
1/2 bunch	parsley with stems

Heat heavy saucepan, add oil, fish bones, carrot, celery, parsley, peppercorns and lemon peel, add water
Bring to a simmer, cover, turn down the heat, skim off foam
Cook for approx 45 minutes, then strain through muslin or sieve
Use straight away or store in the refrigerator

grilled sardines with lemon

serves 4

1kg/36oz	sardines, fresh (filleted)

marinade
6 tbsp	cold pressed olive oil
1 clove	garlic, finely chopped
1/2 cup	lemon juice
4 tbsp	coriander, chopped
salt and black pepper to taste	

Mix up the marinade
Brush the fish with oil and pourhalf the marinade over fish
Leave for 1 hour
Cook the fish under a hot griller for 3-4 min on each side
Brush with marinade each turn

Serve with the remaining marinade poured over the top and a vegetable salad or a big green salad. Turkish or crusty bread served on the side

HINT TO PREPARE FISH

To descale the fish, use the back of a knife and scrape the scales off
Cut of fins with scissors. Slit along the stomach, remove and discard intestines. Wash well, pat dry and place in ceramic or plastic dish

thai seafood casserole

serves 6

The fish markets or your local market would be the best place for your fresh ingredients to make this dish

2 kg/70oz	seafood, mixed fresh (include white fleshed fish, green prawns and crab)
12	black pepper corns
1	kaffir lime leaf
5 cloves	garlic, finely chopped
5	coriander roots, washed and trimmed
1 cup	coconut cream
4	spring onions, finely sliced
4 fresh	chillis (green), finely sliced (optional)
3	red chillis, finley sliced (optional)
6 stalks	lemon grass, finely sliced
3 cups	coconut milk
4 tbsp	fish sauce (anchovies, water and salt)
3 tbsp	maple syrup

Wash and cut up seafood into bite sized pieces
Use a mortar and pestle to crush coriander, garlic and peppercorns into a paste
Use a vegetable peeler to remove a thin strip of the lime skin to use for later
Squeeze lime juice into a cup
Put coconut cream into heavy based saucepan, slowly bring to boil
Add the paste and simmer for 5 mins
Add spring onions, green chillis, lemon grass, lime rind, coconut milk
Bring back to the boil
Add seafood, stir in fish sauce, lime juice, maple syrup, simmer gently
Remove seafood from pan when cooked, transfer to warm serving dish
Season to taste, adjust the balance between sweet, salty and sour
Ladel enough mixture over seafood to just cover

Serve sprinkled with red chillis (optional)

fresh tuna with beetroot

serves 4

1 kg/36oz	tomatoes, quartered
1 clove	garlic crushed
1 cup	basil leaves, rough cut
2 tbsp	dill, fresh, finely sliced
6	baby beetroots
1	red (luscious) capsicum
4	tuna steaks (150 g/5-6oz each)
1	lemon juiced
cold pressed olive oil for roasting	

Grease shallow baking dish with oil and put in tomatoes

Baste tomatoes with a little oil and salt

Cook for 40 minutes in 180°C/350°F oven

Remove from oven and sprinkle with dill and basil

Set aside to allow flavours to blend

Slice capsicum lengthways into 4 pieces, char under grill until skin blisters and turns black

Then place capsicum in a plastic bag and allow to cool, then you can peel off the skin

Put crushed garlic and some oil onto capsicum

Cook beets in salty boiling water until tender, when cooked cut into quarters, lengthways

Drizzle beets with oil and lemon juice and set aside

Sear tuna steaks in hot fry pan, about one minute each side

Divide ingredients into 4 servings

Pile the beetroots onto plate and top with capsicum and tuna steaks

Add tomatoes

Serve garnished with basil and a garden salad!

squid with savoury rice ❤

serves 4

4 med	squid tubes, cleaned
2 cups	rice cooked
2	onions, chopped
3	cloves garlic, crushed
I tsp	cold pressed olive oil
1/2 cup	chives, chopped
I large	lemon, juiced
I pinch	chilli powder (optional)
I med	red capsicum, chopped
440g/16oz	tomatoes, tinned, chopped
1/2 cup	basil, chopped, fresh
a little extra olive oil	
salt and ground black pepper to taste	

Brown onion and garlic in I tablespoon oil
Add 1/2 can of tomatoes, rice and all other ingredients except chopped basil
Stuff the squid tubes with the rice mixture and lay flat in casserole dish. Retain excess rice mixture
Drizzle extra oil over squid then top with remaining tomato.
Cover dish and cook in a medium oven until tender, about I hour
Test with skewer
Heat and divide remaining rice mixture on to 4 serving plates

Serve, sprinkled with basil. fresh tomato wedges, pitted black olives, sliced cucumber and crusty bread

individual fish cutlets ♥

serves 4

4	white fish cutlets (snapper or similar)
I small	red capsicum
I small	green capsicum
I med	zucchini
I stick	celery
I tsp	cummin, ground
I tsp	ginger, freshly grated
I tsp	dill leaves, chopped
2 tbsp	lemon juice
I tbsp	cold pressed olive oil

salt and ground black pepper to taste
banana leaves or foil for wrapping

Cut vegetables into thin strips. heat oil in pan
Stir in cummin, capsicum, zucchini, celery and dill
Stir and cook for 2 minutes
Place each fish cutlet onto a large sheet of foil, or a leaf
Sprinkle with lemon juice - Divide vegetable mixture over fish
Wrap fish in the foil or banana leaves
Place in medium oven for about 25 minutes or until fish is cooked
Remove foil and serve with small boiled potatoes and a green salad

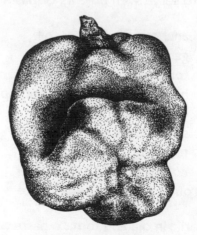

fish steaks with tangy topping ♥

serves 4

Tangy topping can be served either hot or cold.

4	white fish steaks
2	tomatoes, seeded and chopped
4	spring onions, chopped
1 tbsp	basil, chopped
2 tbsp	parsley, chopped
1 tbsp	lemon juice
1 tbsp	cold pressed olive oil
	salt and ground black pepper to taste

Cook fish under grill, 4 to 5 minutes each side. Keep warm until serving
Combine all other ingredients in bowl to make tomato mixture

Serve fish topped with tomato mixture, on a bed of rice or noodles and a big green salad

anchovy sauce

serves 4

A fairly thick sauce to serve with polenta or pasta

1 small tin	anchovy flat fillets + oil
2 cloves	garlic, crushed
1 tbsp	tomato paste
6 tbsp	basil and parsley freshly chopped, more if desired
1	onion, chopped
1 + 1/2 cup	stock, chicken or vegetable
400g/14oz	tomatoes, chopped
2 tbsp	cold pressed olive oil
	sea salt and ground black pepper to taste

Brown onion and garlic in oil, add tomato paste cook for 3 min
Add anchovies and their oil, tomatoes, stock and herbs
Cook until the anchovies have disappeared, approximately 20 minutes

grilled atlantic salmon with mash

serves 4

3	red capsicums cored, cut into quarters
1 tbsp	balsamic vinegar or lemon juice
2 tbsp	cold pressed olive or canola oil
220g /8oz	Atlantic salmon, fillets (4 fillets)
4	tomatoes cut in half
freshly ground black pepper	

mashed potatoes

600g/21oz	potatoes, peeled, quartered
2 tbsp	cold pressed olive or canola oil
1/3 cup	rice, oat or soy milk
2 tbsp	horseradish

Preheat oven to 180°C./350°F
Place capsicums and tomatoes in baking dish
Cover with oil and balsamic vinegar
Add pepper and bake for 30 minutes
Cook salmon under preheated grill for approx 4-5 minutes each side
Cook potatoes until soft and drain
In a pot mash potatoes with milk and oil and stir in the horseradish
Spoon mashed potatoes and roasted capsicums and tomatoes (with juices) onto warmed plates, top with salmon

Serve with a garden salad

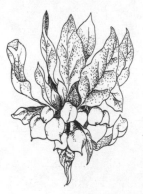

chilli and lime snapper

serves 4

2 tbsp	cold pressed oil
2 tbsp	ginger, grated
1 tbsp	fish sauce
2 tsp	rice syrup or brown sugar
2 tbsp	lime juice
2 tbsp	sweet chilli sauce
2 cloves	garlic crushed
2 bunches	baby bok choy, separate leaves and wash
4	snapper fillets washed
1 cup	coriander leaves washed, fresh
steamed jasmin or basmati rice	

Combine chilli sauce, lime juice, oil, sweetener, ginger, garlic and fish sauce
Add all but 2 tablespoons of mixture to a wok and bring to the boil.
Add bok choy, cover and cook
Stir until leaves are bright green and stalks feel tender (around 2 minutes)
Remove from heat and keep warm
Brush the fish fillets with the left over lime juice mixture
Grill for 2 to 3 minutes on each side

Serve fish sprinkled with coriander leaves on a bed of rice
Place bok choy on the side of the rice

pasta verdi

serves 2 - 4

This pasta dish is made with fresh green herbs and gives you a mineral and vitamin boost to boot!
You need a food processor for putting ingredients in directly

10 sprigs	chives fresh
2 handfulls	flat leaf parsley
1 bunch	basil
10	rocket leaves
1 handful	dill fresh
4	anchovies
1 tbsp	capers
2 cloves	garlic
1/2 cup	pine nuts
1 packet	pasta of your choice
olive oil for blending	

Prepare a large saucepan with enough water to boil your pasta
Place on the heat
Put 1\2 cup olive oil into food processor (you can use less)
Add remaining ingredients, blend until greens are pureéd
If you need more oil add it now
There should be enough oil to create a sauce
The pasta sauce is now done you simply have to wait until the pasta is cooked (normally 10 minutes)

Serve pasta in a big bowl and stir sauce through it for a flavoursome treat!

meat

Some people may be surprised to find recipes including red meat in a book that advocates healthy eating for the liver and bowels. Many people today believe that red meat is unhealthy because it contains saturated fat and is a very concentrated source of animal protein. Others believe that red meat is higher in bacteria than plant food and some avoid it for philosophical reasons. Provided red meat is very fresh and is thoroughly cooked it does not present any greater risk of bowel infection than eating chicken or seafood.

The decision to eat red meat is an individual one and it has been proven categorically that it is not necessary to eat red meat to be healthy or indeed to obtain first class protein.

I have included some recipes containing red meat to cater for those that really enjoy it and cannot live without it. Many women have families to cook for and their husbands and children may demand red meat dishes. It is important to encourage your family to follow the principles of a liver and bowel healthy diet, without making them feel deprived or unhappy. It is just too difficult to have to cook two different meals to fulfill your own dietary requirements and that of your other family members. For these reasons we have included some healthy red meat dishes, that can be prepared in a liver friendly manner, and served with liver cleansing foods to support the liver to process animal meats. We encourage you to use only fresh lean cuts of meat and preferably meat that is organically raised. Make sure that you remove all the fat from the meat and discard any fatty juices after cooking. Always cook the meat very well so that the middle of the meat is cooked thoroughly, as this will kill bacteria. Do not eat meats that are preserved or smoked and make sure that you buy only the freshest meat available. Generally speaking it is best to reduce red meat dishes to no more than once a week.

curried beef and beans ❤

serves 4

500g/18oz	lean beef (preferably rump), cubed
440g/16oz	tomatoes, canned
440g/16oz	barlotti beans,canned, drained
1 large	onion, chopped
1 tsp	red curry paste (more if desired)
1 tbsp	garlic, crushed
1 dstsp	ginger, freshly grated
1 tsp	chilli, fresh, diced, no seeds (optional)
1 tsp	tumeric
1/2 large	lemon, juiced
2 tbsp	mint, freshly chopped
1 tsp	garam masala
2 tbsp	cold pressed olive oil

Brown beef cubes in hot oil until tender, set aside
Sauté onion, garlic and ginger
Add all other ingredients except beans and simmer for 3 minutes
Stir in beef and beans
Cover pan and simmer for 3 to 5 minutes

Serve with cooked brown rice, steamed greens and carrots
Taste to season before serving

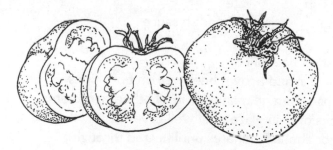

a quick beef & mushroom casserole ❤

serves 4 - 6

750g/27oz	lean beef strips (rump is ideal)
I large	onion, cut into rings
I tbsp	cold pressed olive oil
I med	red capsicum, seeded + chopped
I50g/5oz	field mushrooms
2 cups	water
2 tbsp	tomato paste
2 tsp	oregano, fresh

Heat oil in large pan, brown beef, onion and capsicum, stir often
Add all other ingredients, cover pan, Simmer for about 40 to 45 minutes

Served with rice, steamed carrots, snow peas and a big green salad

sweet mustard glazed beef ❤

serves 4

4	lean porterhouse or scotch fillets
I dstsp	cold pressed olive oil
1/4 cup	brown sugar
1/2 cup	balsamic vinegar
1/4 cup	seeded mustard
1/3 cup	water
I tsp	horseradish sauce

Trim all fat off beef fillets
Heat oil in pan and brown beef well on both sides
Remove pan from heat and stir in all other ingredients
Turn steaks over in glaze until well covered
Simmer for about 5 minutes until heated through
Sprinkle chopped chives or spring onions over rice and vegetables

Served with rice, steamed broccoli, cauliflower and carrot

piquant lamb steaks ❤

serves 4

4	lamb fillets or leg steaks
2 tbsp	natural soy yoghurt
2 tsp	horseradish sauce
I tsp	hot chilli sauce
I tsp	capers, drained and chopped
I small	onion, chopped
I tsp	honey
I tbsp	garlic chives, chopped

a little cold pressed olive oil for browning meat.

Heat oil in pan and cook lamb for 3 minutes on each side
Mix all other ingredients together, spread on each side of lamb
Cook for a further 5 minutes on each side or until tender

Serve with steamed baby potatoes sprinkled with chopped garlic chives,
steamed zucchini and snow peas

spicy beef with pulses ❤

serves 4 or more

500g/18oz	premium fat free minced beef
3 cloves	garlic, crushed (more if desired)
I large	onion, chopped
420g/15oz	tomatoes, canned, chopped
I tsp	chilli (optional)
I tsp	allspice
420g/15oz	chick peas, canned, drained
I tbsp	cold pressed olive oil

Heat oil in pan and brown meat, Add onion and garlic, cook for I minute
Add tomatoes, chilli, allspice and simmer until meat is tender
Stir in chick peas until heated through

Serve on cooked noodles with crusty bread and tossed salad

masala lamb curry ❤

serves 6

Flavour improves if made 1 - 2 days ahead and refrigerated

2 kg/70oz	leg of lamb boned, fat removed, cubed
1/4 cup	cold pressed olive oil
2 large	onions, chopped
4 large	tomatoes, chopped
1/2 cup	water or stock
1/2 cup	coriander, fresh, chopped

masala paste
Blend or process all ingredients until smooth.

1/2 cup	coriander, fresh
1/2 cup	mint, fresh
4 cloves	garlic, crushed
1 tsp	ginger, grated
1/2 tsp	garam masala
1/2 tsp	chilli, fresh, diced (optional)
1/2 tsp	ground cardamon
1/4 cup	apple cider vinegar

Heat oil in large pan
Brown single layers of lamb at a time until browned all over
Brown onion
Add tomatoes and blended masala paste, cover
Reduce heat and simmer for 45 minutes or until lamb is tender

Serve on a bed of rice with blanched spinach and a big green salad

sweets, treats & cakes

For those who wish to reduce both calories and sugar intake in their diets, it is a good idea to reduce the amounts of sweeteners in these recipes. Feel free to experiment with this to suit your individual metabolism.

oatmeal pie crust ♥

For sweet filling add 1 tablespoon honey to mixture.
For savoury filling add salt or herbs to your taste.

2 cups	rolled oats
1 cup	hot water
1/2 cup	rice flour
1 tbsp	cold pressed olive oil
1 tbsp	lemon juice
2 tbsp	LSA

Mix oats and water, bring to the boil in saucepan
Add LSA and stir constantly until mixture thickens
Stand until cold - Fold in other ingredients
Press mixture into a pie dish (20 - 23 cm/10 inches) or 2 small pie dishes

soy custard

serves 2 - 4

2 cups	scalded soy milk
1 tsp	cold pressed olive oil
2	eggs
1/4 cup	maple syrup
1/2 tsp	vanilla

Heat soy milk (a heavy soy like Vitasoy) and beat in the oil
Beat eggs until frothy and gently beat in the maple syrup
While beating, add hot milk in a thin stream. Add vanilla
Pour the mixture into a greased baking dish
Place in shallow pan of water
Bake at 160°C/300°F for 40 minutes until custard is set

banana pops ❤

Cool and delicious on a hot day
Large strawberries can be prepared the same way.

2	passionfruit pulp
I cup	soy natural yoghurt
4	bananas, ripe but firm
chopped nuts or LSA to sprinkle	

Peel bananas, cut in half
Push a pop stick or bamboo skewer through centre of banana
Place in freezer and freeze
Mix passionfruit with soy natural yoghurt and dip frozen banana in
mixture until covered, allow to drip drain
Sprinkle with chopped nuts or LSA and return to freezer

berry surprise ❤

serves 4

I cup	raspberries, blackberries, loganberries, fresh
I tbsp	honey
I	orange, juice and rind grated
2 tsp	gelatine, dissolved in a little hot water (or agar agar)
I cup	soy natural yoghurt

Warm berries, honey, rind and juice, add gelatine mixture
Cool
Gently fold yoghurt through berry mixture
Place in 4 individual serving dishes.
Chill in refrigerator

Serve, garnish with a few extra berries, sliced kiwi fruit and a small scoop
of soy icecream

rockmelon pops ❤

1	rockmelon
1 cup	soy natural yoghurt
1/2 cup	pineapple in natural juice, drained or fresh, diced
1 tsp	mint, fresh, finely chopped
chopped nuts or LSA for sprinkles	

Peel and de-seed half a rockmelon
Cut into wedges similar size to half a banana
Place a popstick or bamboo skewer into fruit wedges
Freeze
Mix all these ingredients together
Dip frozen rockmelon into mixture until covered, allow to drip drain
Sprinkle with chopped nuts or LSA

confetti rice ❤

serves 4

1 cup	oat, soy or rice milk
1 tbsp	honey
1/2 cup	dried apricots, chopped
1/2 cup	natural sultanas
2 slices	mango, dried, chopped
1 + 1/2 cups	rice cooked until tender

Place fluffy rice into a saucepan with other
Mix all together over a low heat until well combined
If necessary, add milk to gain your preferred consistency

Serve warm or cold with a small scoop of soy or vitari ice cream
If left to stand, add more milk as dried fruit will take up the moisture

next best cream ❤

serves 4

A non-dairy gluten free cream, great on desserts, tarts, cakes etc.

1 carton	silken tofu
1 cup	soy milk
1 dstsp	honey
1/2 tsp	pure vanilla essence
3 tbsp	arrowroot

Blend arrowroot with a little milk in a saucepan
Add remaining milk
Stir continually over medium heat until mixture thickens
Allow to cool, Add all other ingredients to thickened mixture
Beat with an electric mixer on low speed until mixture is thick
Will resemble whipped cream

american pumpkin pie ❤

serves 4

2 cups	pumpkin (butternut/blue) cook, mash, drain
1 cup	soft tofu
1 + 1/2 tsp	cinnamon
1/2 tsp	ground ginger or freshly grated
1/2 tsp	ground nutmeg
1/4 cup	soy or oat milk
1/2 cup	honey
1 tbsp	orange rind, grated
1/2 cup	pecans or walnuts, chopped

Blend all ingredients except nuts in a food processor until smooth
Pour mixture into 23 cm (9 inch) pie dish lined with uncooked pie crust,
Sprinkle top with nuts
Bake in moderate oven 35 to 40 minutes until golden and set
Garnish with any fresh fruit, kiwi fruit looks great
Serve with next best cream or soy ice cream

chewy fruit bars ♥

Keeps well in an airtight container. Flavour improves after a day or two.

3/4 cup	honey
I cup	wholemeal plain flour
I tsp	baking powder
1/2 cup	coconut
I cup	fruit medley
5	weetbix, crushed
I	egg lightly beaten
1/2 cup	cold pressed olive oil

Combine all dry ingredients, add egg, oil, honey and mix well
Press mixture over base of lined tin
Cook in moderate oven for about 30 minutes until golden
Cut into small bars when cold

quick mix coconut cake ♥

2 cup	SR wholemeal flour
I cup	raw sugar
I cup	coconut milk, tinned
3/4 cup	cold pressed olive oil
3	eggs
I tbsp	honey
1/4 cup	shredded coconut

Mix all ingredients in a large bowl, beat for 2 to 3 minutes, until the consistency of batter
Pour mixture into a 23cm (9 inches) cake tin lined with greaseproof paper
Bake at 180°C/350°F for about 40 to 45 minutes - test with a skewer
When cool sprinkle with coconut

AUDREY TEA HINT
When the cake is cold cut it into 3 bars, wrap 1 or 2 bars and freeze for later. When defrosting frozen cake slice while still firm as it thaws more quickly.

carrot and apple cake ❤

1 cup	wholemeal SR flour
1/2 cup	honey or maple syrup
3/4 cup	pecans or walnuts chopped
1 cup	carrot, grated
1 cup	granny smith apple grated, leave on skin
2 tbsp	cocoa
1/2 tsp	bicarb soda
2	eggs

Sift flour, cocoa and soda into large bowl
Mix in beaten eggs and all other ingredients and combine well
Spoon mixture into a greased ring tin
Bake in a moderate oven for 40 - 45 minutes or until cooked
Test with a skewer, cool in tin

Serve dusted with a little cinnamon

light and lovely bananas ❤

serves 4

4 large	bananas, peeled, sliced lengthways then crosswise
1 cup	orange juice, freshly squeezed
1/2 cup	lemon juice, freshly squeezed
1 tbsp	orange rind or zest
2 tbsp	honey
1 tsp	cinnamon
3	passion fruit (pulp only)

Place juices, honey and rind in a large flat pan, heat until it simmers, add cinnamon, then add sliced bananas and cook for 1 to 2 minutes
Remove immediately to serving comport
Spoon over juices and top with passionfruit

tangy and spicey apple bake❤

serves 4

2 large	green apples, peeled and cored
3 tbsp	lemon or orange juice
1 tsp	lemon or orange rind, grated
2 tbsp	honey
1 tbsp	raisins or natural sultanas
8	dried apricots
8	prunes, pitted
1/2 tsp	cinnamon, ground

Slice apples into thin wedges
Toss in juice, arrange wedges around the edge of a casserole dish
Combine the juices with the rind, honey and dried fruits
Sprinkle through the cinnamon
Place this mixture through the centre of the casserole
Cover with foil
Bake in a moderate oven for 30 minutes or until apple is tender
Serve warm topped with soy yoghurt or vitari ice cream

This dish can be prepared a few hours ahead, warm before serving

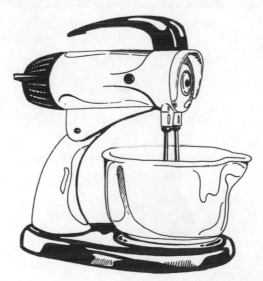

baked winter fruit salad ❤

serves 6.

2 large	green apples, peeled and thinly sliced
2 large	pears, peeled and thinly sliced
I tsp	cinnamon, ground
2 tbsp	honey
1/2 cup	raisins, seeded
1/2 cup	almonds, blanched and sliced
I tbsp	orange peel , shredded
I small tin	crushed pineapple, drained, keep juice

Mix together pineapple, honey, raisins, cinnamon and peel
Place 1/3 of apples and pears overlapping, in a deep 23cm (9 inch) pie dish
Top with 1/2 of the mixture
Place another 1/3 layer of apple and pear slices
Finish with the apple and pear layer
Pour remaining juice over the fruit.
Cover dish and bake in a moderate oven for 45 minutes
Remove cover, shake a little extra cinnamon over top
Scatter the almond slices

Serve warm with natural soy yoghurt and mixed berry vitari ice cream

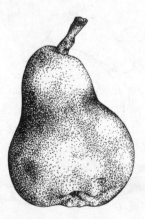

orange and coconut cookies ♥

1 tbsp	tahini
1/4 cup	cold pressed grapeseed oil
3/4 cup	honey
1 large	egg, beaten
2 tbsp	orange juice
1 dstsp	orange rind, grated
1+1/2 cups	stoneground wholemeal SR flour
1/2 cup	shredded coconut
1 + 1/4 cups	LSA

Mix tahini, oil and honey together until smooth
Stir in beaten egg, juice and rind
Add coconut, LSA and flour and combine all together
Roll teaspoonful into a ball
Flatten on tray
Bake at 180°C/350°F for 12 - 15 minutes, until golden brown

berry mousse

serves 4

2 cups	berries, strawberries, raspberries
5 tsp	agar agar flakes
1 tsp	tahini
1	egg white (room temp)
1+1/2 cups	apple juice
1/2 cup	tofu
1/4 cup	maple syrup

Wash berries, if strawberries are large cut in halves
Combine agar agar and apple juice in a saucepan and bring to boil
Turn down heat and simmer till agar agar has dissolved
Combine berries, liquid, tofu, tahini and blend till smooth
Heat maple syrup, boil for 6 min until a caramel like texture
Beat egg white to form peaks, still beating, drip in hot maple syrup
Fold egg white into berry mixture
Place in serving dishes and chill

fruit loaf ❤

Store in an airtight container.

I cup	rice bran
I cup	dark brown sugar
I cup	soy milk
125g/5oz	dried apricots, chopped or mixed dried fruits
I tbsp	honey
I cup	stoneground wholemeal SR flour
I tbsp	sesame or sunflower seeds

Mix together rice bran, milk, sugar, honey and fruit
Let stand for 10 minutes
Stir in flour until blended
Place mixture in oiled loaf tin, sprinkle top with seeds
Bake in a moderate oven for about I hour
Test with skewer before removing to a cooling rack

pear truffles ❤

Serve these with coffee after a leisurely dinner

I cup	pears, dried
3/4 cup	raisins
I tsp	preserved ginger (more if desirable)
2 tbsp	honey
I tbsp	LSA
I cup	coconut, toasted

Mince dried fruit and ginger
Combine in a bowl with honey, LSA and 1/2 of the coconut. Mix well
Form mixture into small balls and roll in the remaining coconut
Slightly flatten to form thick button shapes
Refrigerate until firm then store in fridge in an airtight container
Can be made several days ahead

fruity petit fours ♥

I cup	dried pears, chopped
1/2 cup	dried apricots, chopped
1/2 cup	cashews, chopped
1/2 cup	shredded coconut
I tbsp	lemon juice
I tbsp	honey
425ml/15oz	coconut cream

Mix all ingredients together with enough coconut cream to bind the mixture

Stand covered for I hour

If mixture is too dry add more coconut cream to hold it together and make it pliable

Roll into small balls, press a cashew nut into top of each ball

Place in small confectionery paper patty cups

Cover and store in fridge in an airtight container

fruit chews ♥

Must be stored in the refrigerator.

I cup	nut paste (almond, macadamia, or cashew nut)
3 cups	rice bubbles (any rice cereal)
1/2 cup	honey
1/4 cup	raw sugar
1/2 cup	sultanas
1/2 cup	currants
I tsp	vanilla essence

Combine nut paste, honey and sugar in large saucepan

Stir over a low heat until mixture is dissolved

Add remaining ingredients and mix until everything is well coated

Press firmly into a grease-proof paper lined tin 28 x 18cm (11 x 7 inch)

Refrigerate for I hour

Cut into thin small fingers

sinful cake ❤

Great for visitors

2+ 1/2 cups	wholmeal plain flour
1/3 cup	cocoa powder
1 cup	raw sugar
1 + 1/2 cups	walnuts & brazil, chopped
1/4 cup	LSA or LAA
1 cup	zucchini grated
1 cup	carrot grated
1 cup	cold pressed olive oil
400g/14oz	pears, (drained), or poached yourself
4	eggs beaten
1 tsp	baking powder
1 tsp	cinnamon
1 tsp	bicarb soda

Sift all dry ingredients into a large bowl
Make a well and add all other ingredients - Mix well
Pour mixture into square tin lined with greaseproof paper
Bake at 180°C/350°F for about 1 hour or until cooked
Test with a skewer. Cool in tin

PLEASE NOTE:
All wholemeal SR and plain flour can be substituted with other flours. For recipes that need SR flour use 1 teaspoon of baking powder plus the other flour. A combination of buckwheat and soy flour, or rice, buckwheat and soy flour, works well and is gluten free. Using different flours will change the consistancy of your cake or loaf, however it will still be delicious. When plain flour is needed omit the baking powder.

fruit and nut salad ❤

serves 6 - 8

I	red apple diced, skin on, core out
I	green apple diced, skin on, core out
I cup	celery, diced
I	avocado diced, skin off, stone out
I	red onion in thin half rings
425g/15oz	unsweetened pineapple pieces, retain juice, or fresh
I cup	parsley, chopped
I cup	pecans or walnuts, chopped

Gently toss apples and avocado in pineapple juice, drain
Mix with all other ingredients.
Dress with no 3 dressing (see page 192)

peachy treats ❤

serves 6 to 8

Made in a flash, this dessert is light and very tasty
Peach or pear halves can be used

825g/30oz	peach halves, drained or 6 - 8 fresh peaches
100g/3-4oz	natural soy yoghurt
I cup	mixed dried fruit, chopped
I tbsp	apple or orange juice
I pinch	ground cinnamon
1/2 cup	toasted coconut

Arrange peach halves in individual serving dishes
Mix fruit juice with dried fruit
Stand for about 1/2 hour, then fold into yoghurt
Spoon mixture into hollows of peaches, sprinkle with cinnamon
Top each serve with coconut

baked bread custard ♥

serves 6

4 large	eggs
3 cups	soy milk
1/2 cup	raw sugar
1/2 cup	coconut
3 - 4 slices	fruit loaf, (see page 272)
2 tbsp	jam of your choice (sugarless)
1/2 tsp	vanilla essence
1/2 tsp	ground nutmeg or cinnamon

Spread fruit loaf with jam and cut into pieces
Place in a 2 litre/70oz capacity ovenproof dish
Beat eggs with sugar, stir in vanilla and coconut, pour over fruit loaf and sprinkle with spices
Place dish in a baking pan with about 2.5cm (1 inch) of hot water
Bake at 160°C/300°F and bake for around 1 hour until custard is set

basic pastry

2 tbsp	gelatine or agar agar
1/2 tsp	bicarbonate soda
1/2 cup	water
1/2 cup	cold pressed olive oil
1/2 tsp	salt
1/2	lemon, juiced
200g/7oz	potato and chick pea flour
50g/2oz	rice flour
50g/2oz	arrowroot

Preheat the oven to 180°C/350°F, dissolve gelatine in hot water
Put gelatine, lemon and oil into a large ceramic bowl
Sift flours, salt and bicarb into the oil and gelatine mixture
Mix the dough until it pulls away from the side and forms a ball
Place onto a board, wrap between the plastic
Roll out between 2 sheets of plastic, to desired thickness, discard plastic
When handling the dough, rub a small amount of oil on your hands
Bake in oven for approx 15 minutes, until golden brown

goodness galore ♥

This cake is unbelievably tasty, nutritious and energy boosting.
Store in an airtight container

I cup	natural sultanas
I cup	dates, chopped
I cup	dried apricots, chopped
I cup	brazil nuts, chopped
I cup	sunflower seeds
1/4 cup	LSA
1/4 cup	sesame seeds
I tsp	mixed spice
2	eggs, beaten
2 cups	wholemeal SR flour
2 cups	orange juice, fresh

Place all ingredients except the flour and eggs into a large saucepan
Bring slowly to the boil, stirring continually, simmer for 3 to 5 minutes
Cool, then stir in eggs and flour
Place in paper lined cake tin
Bake in a slow oven at about 150°C/300°F for 1 hour or until cooked
when tested with a skewer
Cool in tin

HINT TO MAKE NUT MILK

To make one cup of nut milk mix one cup of hot water or fruit juice with
two tablespoons of any nut butter such as hazel nut, Brazil nut, cashew
nut, or almond and mix in a blender until smooth.

fruits and flakes biscuits ♥

Store in airtight container.

5 cups	cornflakes
1 cup	coconut
1/4 cup	linseeds, ground
1/2 cup	raw sugar
1 cup	natural sultanas
1 cup	dates, chopped
1 cup	wholemeal SR flour
3/4 cup	cold pressed olive oil
2	eggs, lightly beaten

Combine all dry ingredients in a large bowl, add oil and eggs
Mix well
Take heaped dessertspoons of mixture, shape into rounds
Press lightly with hand
Place on an oiled oven tray about 2.5cm (1 inch) apart
Bake in a moderate oven for about 10 minutes until golden brown
Leave on tray for a few minutes
Place on a wire rack to cool

AUDREY TEA HINT
If you slightly warm oil and honey in a small saucepan it will mix through the
dry ingredients more easily.

honey chews 💜

1 cup	rolled oats
1 cup	sultanas or mixed fruit
1/2 cup	wholemeal SR flour
1/2 cup	raw sugar
1/2 cup	coconut
1/2 cup	cold pressed olive oil
1 tbsp	honey
2 dstsp	orange rind grated

Combine all ingredients together until the mixture clings
Press evenly into a lined tin, 28 x 18cm (11 x 7 inch)
Bake in a moderate oven for 15 to 20 minutes until golden brown
Cut into small bars while still hot, remove from tin when cold

muesli slice 💜

2 cups	muesli with the lot
1/2 cup	wholemeal SR flour
1/4 cup	sesame seeds
1/2 cup	cold pressed olive oil
1/4 cup	peanut paste (or hazelnut, almond, cashew etc.)
1/4 cup	honey
1 + 1/4 cup	raw sugar

In a saucepan stir oil, peanut paste (or similar), honey and sugar over a low
heat until combined. Cool
In a large bowl mix all other ingredients together
Add liquid mixture and combine well
Spread mixture evenly in paper lined tray 20 x 30cm (8 x 12 inch)
Bake in a moderate oven for about 20 minutes or until lightly browned
Cool in pan before cutting into squares with a sharp knife
Store cold in an airtight container

spicy apple fruit cake ♥

1/2 cup	cold pressed oil
1/4 cup	apple juice
1 cup	brown sugar
1	egg
1/2 cup	walnuts, chopped
500g/18oz	mixed dried fruits
3 med	apples, peeled and grated
2 cups	wholemeal SR flour
2 tsp	bi-carb soda
1/2 tsp	nutmeg, mixed spice, ginger and cinnamon

Beat together egg and sugar
Add oil and apple juice and mix well
Add fruit, apple and nuts
Combine well, add sifted flour, soda and spices
Place mixture in a large loaf or square lined tin
Bake about 1 hour in a moderate oven
Test with skewer

carob fruit loaf ♥

No eggs, sugar or fat

1 cup	mixed dried fruit
1 cup	wheatgerm
1 + 1/2 cups	oat, soy or rice milk
1/4 cup	carob powder
1 cup	wholemeal SR flour

Place fruits, wheatgerm and milk in a large bowl
Cover and let stand for 2 hours
Fold in sifted carob and flour and mix well
Place in lined loaf tin and bake at 180°C/350°F for 45 to 60 minutes

tangy fruit loaf ❤

1/4 cup	cold pressed oil
1/2 cup	brown sugar
1	egg
3	bananas, sliced
1/2 cup	dates, chopped
1 + 1/2 cups	wholemeal SR flour
1/2 cup	wheatgerm
1/2 tsp	bi-carb soda
1/2 cup	pecan, brazil or walnuts, chopped
1	lemon, juice

Heat oil and sugar in saucepan and stir until sugar dissolves
Add egg and beat well, stir in bananas, dates, nuts and lemon juice
Add sifted flour, wheatgerm and soda
Fold in and blend well
Pour into greased loaf tin
Bake in a moderate oven for about 1 hour

banana cake ❤

250g/9oz	wholemeal SR flour
1/2 cup	cold pressed oil
125g/4-5oz	raw sugar or honey (or less if desired)
2 large	ripe bananas, mashed
3 tbsp	soy or rice milk
1 tsp	bi-carb soda
1 tsp	vanilla
2	eggs

Beat oil and sugar until smooth, add eggs, beat well
Add mashed bananas, mix milk, soda and vanilla together
Add alternately with sifted flour until all ingredients are folded smoothly together
Place mixture in a lined cake tin
Sprinkled with cinnamon or chopped walnuts
Cook in a moderate oven for about 45 minutes, test with skewer
Cool in tin for 10 minutes before removing to a cooling rack

poached fruitee pears ♥

serves 4 or more

3 large	pears, peeled and cored
1/2 cup	dried apricots, chopped
1/2 cup	shredded coconut
1/4 cup	almonds, chopped
1/2 tsp	cinnamon
1 tsp	honey (more if desired)
1 cup	apple or apricot juice

Cut pears in half and lay centre-up in a casserole dish
In a bowl mix together apricots, coconut, almonds and cinnamon
Add enough honey to bind the mixture together
Divide the mixture evenly over the six pear halves
Add one cup of juice to casserole, pour gently over the fruit
Cover and bake in preheated oven at 180°C/350°F, approx 30 minutes

Serve barely warm, with frozen apple and pear dessert

fruit and nut energy bars ♥

Stores well in an airtight container

1 + 1/2 cups	wholemeal SR flour
1 cup	raw sugar
1/2 cup	cold pressed olive oil
1 cup	dates, chopped
1 cup	walnuts, chopped
2 tbsp	maple syrup

Rub flour and all other dry ingredients together in a large bowl
Put oil and maple syrup in a saucepan
Stir over low heat until melted and combined
Cool and mix into dry ingredients
Place in lined square cake tin, 23cm (9 inch)
Bake in a moderate oven for about 30 minutes or until golden brown
Cut into bars with sharp knife while still warm

apple and pear ice cream ♥
a non dairy dessert

serves 4

1	pear, stem removed, skin on
1	granny smith apple, skin on
1/2 cup	soy milk
1 tsp	honey
1 small scoop	Vitari ice cream
1 tbsp	gelatine, or agar agar
425ml/15oz	coconut milk

Mix all ingredients together in a food processor until smooth
Pour into a container of your choice and freeze
Serve in scoops with crushed almonds or with poached pears

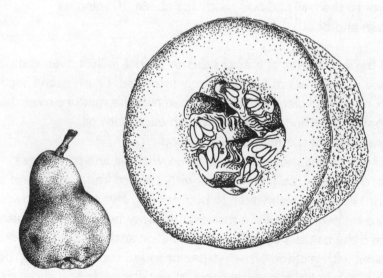

AUDREY TEA HINT
Any recipe that has a bran type cereal content can have a wonderful added
flavour if you substitute the same amount of LSA mixture.

baklava

Makes about 30 pieces

1+3/4 cup	cold pressed olive oil
500g/18oz	filo pastry (fresh or frozen)
2 cups	walnuts, finely chopped
1 cup	almonds, finely chopped
2 tsp	cinnamon, ground
1/4 tsp	cloves, ground
1/2 cup	brown sugar, (optional)

syrup

2 cups	water
2+1/2 cups	honey (or 2 cups brown sugar + 2 tbsp honey)
3 whole	cloves
1 stick	cinnamon
1 tbsp	lemon juice
thin strip of lemon rind	

for the syrup
Place all ingredients into a saucepan, stir over heat until dissolved
Bring to the boil and boil gently for about 10 minutes
Strain and cool

Oil base and sides of a 33x23x5cm/13x9x2 inches oven dish
Place nine sheets of filo separately into dish, brush each sheet with oil
Mix nuts and spices together, spread half the mixture over the filo
Top with another two sheets, brush each with oil
Spread last of the nut mixture on top
Top with eight sheets, each brushed with oil and trim edges
Score through top layers of filo with a sharp knife - diamond shapes
Sprinkle lightly with water to prevent top layers curling upwards
Bake on centre shelf in a moderately slow oven for 30 minutes
Move the baklava up one shelf, cook for another 30 minutes
Cover with greased brown paper or foil (if top is colouring too quickly)
While the baklava is in the oven, make the syrup and allow to cool
Filo MUST be cooked thoroughly, When cooked take out of the oven
Spoon COOL syrup over HOT baklava
Leave for several hours before cutting right through into serving portions

Appendix Section Three

Conversion Chart for Recipes and Cooking

Ounces	Grams
1	28
2	57
3	85
4	113
5	142
6	170
7	198
8	227
9	255
10	283

For additional amounts select the appropriate conversion above and multiply or add or both.

For example 15 ounces   = 10 ounces (283 grams)
+ 5   ounces (142 grams)   = 15 ounces (425 grams)

Pounds	Kilograms
1	0.45
2	0.91
3	1.36
4	1.81
5	2.27
6	2.72
7	3.17
8	3.63
9	4.10
10	4.54

Farenheit (°F)	Centigrade (°C)
200	93
250	121
300	149
350	177
400	204

For other temperature conversions use the following formula:

F to C : subtract 32, then divide by 1.8
C to F : multiply by 1.8, then add 32

KITCHEN MEASURES

Measure	Ounces	Millilitres
One teaspoon	0.17	5
One tablespoon	0.5	14
One cup	8	227
One pint	16	454
One quart	32	908
One gallon	128	3632

HELPFUL CONVERSION CHART

Ounces to millilitres:
multiply ounce figure by 30 to get number of millilitres
Pounds to kilograms:
multiply pound figure by 0.45 to get number of kilograms
Pounds to grams:
multiply pound figure by 453 to get number of grams
Grams to ounces:
multiply gram figure by .0353 to get number of ounces
Ounces to grams:
multiply ounce figure by 28.3 to get number of grams
One teaspoon = 5 grams
Three teaspoons = one tablespoon = 1/2 ounce = 14.3 grams
Two tablespoons = one ounce = 28.35 grams
Agar-agar (1 bar) = 4-6 tablespoons agar-agar flakes
Garlic concentrated (1 teaspoon) = 2 cloves fresh garlic
Herbs, dried (1/4 teaspoon) = 2 tablespoons fresh herbs

SWEETENERS EQUIVALENTS

1/2 cup sweetener =
- 1/2 cup maple syrup
- 1/2 cup coconut sugar
- 1/2 cup raw sugar
- 1/3 cup molasses
- 1/2 cup honey
- 1 + 1/2 cups barley malt extract
- 1/2 cup fruit juice concentrate
- 1/2 cup fruit juice
- 1/2 cup unsweetened frozen juice concentrate

Organic Food Sources and Control

Growers who are inspected regularly by one of the Independent Certification Bodies produce the foods that are certified as organic.

USA

Internatinal Federation of Organic Agricultural Movements (IFOAM)
Suite 15/118, 1st Avenue South, Jamestown ND USA 58401
Email: IFOAM@+/online.de

The Organic Trade Association
PO Box 1078, Greenfield, MA 01302
Phone: (413) 774 5484 Fax: (413) 774 6432

Sustain, The Environmental Information Group
920 N. Franklin, Suite 206, Chicago, IL 60610
Phone: (312) 951 8999   Fax: (312) 951 5696

UK

Christopher Argent/Steve Holmes (S&C Meats)
259 Shay Lane, Holmfield, Halifax HX2 9AG
Email: info@organic-meat.co.uk

Artificial Sweeteners

During my widespread travels I am continually shocked by the large number of people still consuming artificial sweeteners, especially the highly toxic sweetener, aspartame. These artificial sweeteners must be broken down by the detoxification systems in the liver and increase the workload of the liver much more than natural sugars.

If you increase the workload of the liver's detoxification systems, you will use up valuable energy in the liver cells, that is required for fat metabolism. Thus your ability to burn fat will be compromised and you will gain weight more easily. This explains why artificial sweeteners do not help those with weight excess, indeed they are fattening.

Aspartame is a molecule composed of three components—aspartic acid, phenylalanine and methanol. Once broken down by the liver, the methanol (wood alcohol) converts into formaldehyde and formic acid (ant-sting poison). Formaldehyde, a deadly neurotoxin, is a common embalming fluid and a class A carcinogen.
Aspartame is a commonly used artificial sweetener.

Some people have suffered aspartame related disorders with doses as small as that carried in a single stick of chewing gum. Pilots who drink diet sodas may be more susceptible to flicker vertigo, flicker-induced epileptic activity, sudden memory loss, dizziness during instrument flight and gradual loss of vision. Some pilots have experienced grand mal seizures in the cockpits of commercial airline flights and have lost medical certification to fly.

The FDA has received more than 10,000 consumer complaints about artificial sweeteners. That's 80 per cent of all complaints about food additives, yet they remain comatose and have done nothing to alert the American public who assume that since it's so highly advertised, it must be safe.

If you are using aspartame and have headaches, depression, slurred speech, loss of memory, fibromyalgia-type symptoms, loss of sensation in lower legs or shooting pains, loss of equilibrium, vertigo, anxiety attacks, chronic fatigue, vision loss, seizures or heart palpitations, you may have ASPARTAME DISEASE! Many physicians are diagnosing multiple sclerosis (MS) when in reality it is methanol toxicity caused by aspartame which mimics MS.

Researchers at Massachusetts Institute of Technology surveyed 80 people who suffered brain seizures after eating or drinking products with Aspartame. The Community Nutrition Institute states 'These 80 cases meet the FDA's own definition of an imminent hazard to public health, which requires the FDA to expeditiously remove a product from the market'.

Pregnant women or those trying to conceive should avoid artificial sweeteners. Foetal tissue cannot tolerate methanol, and Dr James Bowen calls NutraSweet instant birth control. The foetal placenta can concentrate phenylalanine which may increase the risk of mental retardation. Aspartame tests on animals produced brain and mammary tumors.

During Operation Desert Storm, truckloads of diet drinks cooked in the Arabian sun. Aspartame liberates methanol in the can! Thousands of service men and women returned home with chronic fatigue syndrome and weird toxic symptoms!
Aspartame and other artificial sweeteners make you crave carbohydrates so you gain weight. They do not help diabetics although millions of diabetics are using aspartame products.

Dr H. J. Roberts (world expert on Aspartame and diabetic specialist) says 'I now advise ALL patients with diabetes and hypoglycemia to avoid Aspartame products.'
Neurosurgeon, Russell Blaylock, MD, in his book entitled *EXCITOTOXINS— THE TASTE THAT KILLS*, says Aspartame may trigger clinical diabetes! He states that, 'What really concerns me about aspartame is its association with brain tumors as well as pancreatic, uterine and ovarian tumors and that so many develop an Alzheimer's-like syndrome with prolonged exposure'.

Artificial sweeteners are dangerous toxins in our society because of their ubiquitous presence in thousands of foods, even children's vitamins and medicine and are found on every restaurant table and in every hotel/motel room.

References:
H. J. ROBERTS, MD, FACP, FCCP. Books and publications:Aspartame: is it Safe? The Charles Press, PO Box 15715S, Philadelphia PA 19103.
Much of this information was prepared from facts and statistics collected by the organisation MISSION POSSIBLE, PO BOX 28098, Atlanta, GA 30358 USA. For further information on aspartame e-mail betty@pd.org and put as the subject line 'sendme help'.

Farewell Thoughts

In the Future

Medicine of the next century will be revolutionised by genetic engineering. It will be known as the "Biotech Century" and will give doctors incredible power over thousands of diseases that have previously afflicted and shortened human lives.

The human genome consisting of around 100,000 genes encoded by 3 billion chemical pairs in DNA, will be fully decoded within a matter of years. By tinkering with genes engineers will get more control over the prevention and treatment of cancer, influence the growth of blood vessels, reset the genes that control ageing and create new organs from primitive human cells (stem cells).

Serious diseases cause the death of cells and the more cells that die, the harder it is to replace them. In highly developed organs of the body such as the brain, the cells are so specialised that they cannot duplicate themselves. This is why dementia is so permanent- the brain cells cannot replace themselves and the brain gradually shrinks. The liver in contrast has a reasonable ability to renew damaged and dead liver cells, which is why many types of liver disease are reversible. Once a critical amount of liver cells have died however, it is impossible for this regeneration to take place.

This is where genetic engineering will come into its own because it will allow doctors to take primitive (unspecialised) cells known as stem cells, and direct the way they will grow. For example they could tinker with the stem cell's genes to make it grow into brain cells, pancreas cells, liver cells or whatever was required. This would give patients healthy new replacement tissue, which would not suffer from rejection by the immune system because it contains the same DNA as the host.

Engineers at the University of Wisconsin, USA, have recently isolated these primitive stem cells and channelled them to grow into bone cells, muscle cells and brain cells. This type of designer tissue factory is still in the very early stages with unforeseen problems to overcome, however progress will be rapid.

Another genetic technique involves using a fully developed human cell and resetting its developmental instructions back to a pure state or a clear slate if you like. It is a bit like giving the cell amnesia so it can no longer remember what it was supposed to do. Once that occurs, the engineer gains complete control over that cell's destiny, and can make the cell develop along several different ways. For example it could be used to clone an animal or human into a genetically identical replica of its parent, or it could be turned into healthy body tissues or organs. These could be used to replace diseased organs, such as a liver in the parent of the reset cell.

Even though those of the next century will be very fortunate to be the recipients of this powerful form of curative medicine, they will still need to protect their new organs and cells from the external influences that can recreate disease in healthy new tissue. They will need to nurture their environment, avoid toxic chemicals, practise good hygiene, utilise vaccinations and provide their cells with the essential living nutrients that fuel them.

Next century we will need to see a true merging of new age genetic technology with the ancient wisdom of nutritional, environmental and mind-body-spirit medicine. The human genome is really just a seed, and even if we can make it a perfect seed, without good soil we will still have unforeseen diseases and malformations that can occur along the way.

More than ever before in the course of history, we need to utilize the power of nutritional medicine to chart a safe passage through the chemical waters and atmosphere, that will take us time to repair. Let us hope that time is a luxury we still have.

I hope that you have enjoyed reading this book, and find it of use in your every day life. If you have any suggestions or queries, you may contact the publisher - SCB International Inc. PMB 101, suite 2A, 13910 Nth. Frank Lloyd Wright Blvd. Scottsdale, AZ 85260

Bibliography - References

1. Saint Mary's Thistle

Boari C, et al, Occupational toxic liver diseases. Therapeutic effects of silymarin. Min Med 1985; 72(2):679-88

Floersheim GL et al. Effects of penicillin and silymarin on liver enzymes and blood clotting factors in dogs given a boiled preparation of Amanita phalloides. Toxicology and Applied Pharmacology. 46:455-462, 1978

Valenzuela A. et al. Silybin dihemisuccinate protects rat erythrocytes against phenylhydrazine-induced lipid peroxidation and haemolysis. Planta Medica. 53:402-405,1987.

Valenzuela A. et al. Silymarin protection against hepatic lipid peroxidation induced by acute ethanol intoxication in the rat. Biochemical Pharmacology. 34:2209-2212, 1985.

Kropacova K,et al. Protective and therapeutic effect of Silymarin on the development of latent liver damage. Radiat Biol Radioecol 1998 May;38(3):411-5

Vengerovski AI et al. Liver protective action of silybinene in experimental CCL4 poisoning. Farmakologiya I Toksikologiya. 50:67-69,1987

Wagner H. Antihepatoxic flavonoids. Progress in Clinical and Biology Research. 213:319-331,1986

Flora K, et al. Milk Thistle (Silybum marianum) for the therapy of liver disease. Am. J. Gastroenterol 1998 Feb;93(2):139-43

Salmi HA, et al, Effect of silymarin on chemical, functional and morphological alteration of the liver:a double blind controlled study. Scandinavian J Gastroenterol 1982;17:417-21

2. Selenium

Margaret Rayman, Dietary Selenium: time to act, British Medical Journal Vol. 314, 387, 8th Feb. 1997

Boost Your Energy. Dr. Sandra Cabot, 1997, Women's Health Advisory Service

3. Taurine

Orthoplex Research Bulletin, Taurine the detoxifying amino acid. Nutrients in profile, Henry Osiecki. Bioconcepts Publishing.

Nutrients in Profile, Henry Osiecki, Bioconcepts Publishing. Phone (07)3525088

4. S-adenosyl-L-methionine

Lieber CS. Susceptibility to alcohol-related liver injury. Alcohol 1994;2 Suppl:315-26

5. N-acetyl cysteine (NAC)

Bonkovsky HL. Therapy of hepatitis C: other options. Hepatology 1997 Sep;3(1 Suppl)143S

Beloqui O, et al. N-acetyl cysteine enhances the response to interferon-alpha in chronic hepatitis C. J Interferon Res 1993;13:279-82

6. Liquorice root and Liver disease

Yamamura Y, et al. The relationship between pharmacokinetic behaviour of glycyrrhizin and hepatic function in patients with acute hepatitis and cirrhosis. Biopharm Drug Dispos 1995 Jan;16(1):13-21

Van Rossum TG, et al. Review article:glycyrrhizin as a potential treatment for chronic hepatitis C. Ailment Pharmacol Ther 1998 Mar; 12(3):199-205

7. Liver Function

Parveen J. Kumar BSc, MD, FRCP, Michael L Clark MD, FRCP. Clinical Medicine, 2nd Edition Pg. 237-287, Bailliere Tindall

Bland J.S., Bralley J.A., Nutritional up-regulation of hepatic detoxification enzymes. The Journal of Applied Nutrition, 1992,44; No. 3 & 4

The Physicians Handbook of Clinical Nutrition, Henry Osiecki, Bioconcepts Publishing

The Liver Cleansing Diet Book, Dr Sandra Cabot, W.H.A.S. 1996

Fraser, R., Dobbs, B.R. Rogers, G.W.T.(1995) Lipoproteins and the liver sieve: The role of the fenestrated sinusoidal endothelium in lipoprotein metabolism, atherosclerosis and cirrhosis. Hepatology. 21:863-874

Research on the liver filter (sieve): contact Professor Robin Fraser at Department of Pathology, Christchurch School of Medicine, New Zealand

Buist RA. CFS-Xenobiotic/Toxin Exposure. Int Clin Nutr Rev 1988; 8(4):173-5

Bland JS CFS- Detoxification and Mitochondrial Damage. J Nutr Environ Med 1995;5:255

Jost G et al. Phase 1-Caffeine Test. Hepatology 1987;7(2):338-44

Podolsky DK et al. Phase 11-Major Conjugation Pathways. Harrison's Principles of Internal Medicine. 13th Edition. 1994. McGraw-Hill Inc. NY

James RC et al. Glutathione/Sulphate Conjugation. Toxicol Appl Pharmacol 1993;118:159

8. Cirrhosis

Trotter JF, Brenner DA, Current and prospective therapies for hepatic fibrosis. Compr Ther 1995 Jun;21(6):303-7

Cabre E, Gassull MA. Nutritional support in liver disease. Eur J Gastroenterol Hepatol 1995;7(6):528-32

Corrao G, Ferrari PA. Exploring the role of diet in modifying the effect of known disease determinants: application to risk factors of liver cirrhosis. Am J Epidemiol 1995 Dec 1;142(11):1136-46

9. Vitamin E and Cirrhosis

Von Herbay A, et al. Vitamin E improves the aminotransferase status of patients suffering with viral hepatitis C: a randomized, double-blind, placebo-controlled study. Free Radical Res 1997 Dec;27(6):599-605

10. Olive Leaf Extract

Nature's Antibiotic, Dr. Morton Walker, Kensington Publishing Corp.

Juven, B.,et al. Studies on the mechanism of the antimicrobial action of oleuropein. Journal of Applied Bacteriology 35:559-567, 1972

Elliott, G.A. et al, Preliminary safety studies with calcium elenolate, an antiviral agent. Antimicrobial Agents and Chemotherapy, American Society for Microbiology, 1970

Renis, H.E. Inactivation of myxoviruses by calcium elenolate. Antimicrobial Agents and Chemotherapy pp. 194-199 August 1975

Walker, M. Antimicrobial attributes of olive leaf extract. Townsend Letter for Doctors & Patients, #156, July 1996, pp.80-85

Walker, M. Olive leaf extract: The new oral treatment to counteract most types of pathological organisms. Explore for the Professional 7(4):31-37, Nov. 1996

11. Pantothenate

Arsenio L et al. Effectiveness of long term treatment with pantothenate in patients with dyslipidaemia. Clinical Therapeutics. 8:537-541, 1986

Gaddi A et al. Controlled evaluation of pantothenate : A natural hypolipidaemic compound in patients with different forms of hyperlipoproteinaemia. Atherosclerosis. 50:73-83, 1984.

Watanabe A et al. Lowering of blood acetaldehyde but not ethanol concentration by pantothenate following alcohol ingestion. Alcoholism: Clinical and Experimental Research. 9 (3):272-276,1985

12. Vitamin B 12

Vitamin B 12 confirmed as effective sulphite allergy blocker.
Allergy Observer. 4(2):1, March-April 1987

Beck WS. Vitamin B 12 (Cobalamin) and the nervous system. N. Eng. J. Med. 318:1752-1754, 1988.

Jacobsen DW. et al. Cobalamin protection in sulphite sensitive asthmatics (SSA), Journal of Allergy and Clinical Immunology (Supplement). 73:135, 1984.

13. Folic Acid
Froster-Iskenius U et al. Folic acid treatment in males and females with fragile X syndrome. American Journal of Medical Genetics. 23:272-289, 1986

14. Glutathione
Meister A. Selective modification of glutathione metabolism. Science 220:472-477,1983
The Doctor's Vitamin Encyclopedia, Arrow Books, Dr. Sheldon Hendler. M.D., PhD.

15. Incidence of Liver Disease
American Liver Foundation, 1425 Pompton Ave. Cedar Grove, N.J. 07009 U.S.A.

16. Cholesterol Levels
Lancet, 1992; 339:1168-9

17. Crohn's Disease
Ref. Atkinson, Kent, Dairy Board says no to monitoring milk for Johne's disease, NZPA, 24 Nov. 1997.

18. Brindleberry - Natural Fat Burner
Sullivan A.C. et al. Metabolic Inhibitors of lipid biosynthesis as anti-obesity agents. Biological Pharmacology of Obesity, Elsevier Science Publishers, Amsterdam, 1983, pp.311-325
Roo R.N. et. al. Lipid lowering and anti-obesity effect of Hydroxy Citric Acid. Journal Nutr. Res 1998; 8:209-212

19. Mad Cow Disease
Rhodes, Richard, Deadly Feasts: Tracking the secrets of a terrifying new plague, Simon & Schuster New York 1997.

20. Cow's Milk
http://www.notmilk.com/

21. Aspartame Toxicity
Betty Martini - Email: bettym19@idt.net
Mission Possible - Email: Mission-P-USA@altavista.net
                    Website: www.dorway.com

22. Alpha-lipoic acid
Medical Research Institute, 573 Meadow Road, Aptos CA 95003
Fax: 415 673 9053, Email: www.lipoic.com

SCB International Inc. and W.H.A.S. Directory - International Contact Details

INTERNATIONAL
Web site: http://www.whas.com.au
Web site: http://www.liverdoctor.com
E-mail: cabot@ozemail.com.au

UNITED STATES OF AMERICA

SCB International Inc.
PMB 101, Suite 2A, 13910 N.Frank Lloyd Wright Blvd. Scottsdale, AZ 85260.
Voice-mail: 602-860-4299   Free-Call: 1888-75LIVER
GK Products
10088 NW 3rd Place, Coral Springs, Florida 33071
Phone: 1888-752-4286   Phone: 1888-755-4837   Fax: 954-752-4061
E-mail: ajeet@worldnet.att.net   Web Site: www.gkproducts.com
Ten Speed Press
1201 9th St. Dock W2 Berkley, Ave CA 94710
Phone: 510-559-1600   Free-Call: 1800-841-2665

AUSTRALIA

Health Advisory Service & Womens Health Network
PO Box 54, Cobbitty, New South Wales 2570
Phone: 612-4653-1445   Fax: 612-4653-1144
Dr. Sandra Cabot Health Clinic - Sydney
Phone: 612-93282-900

NEW ZEALAND

Thompsons Nutrition
25 Constellation Dve, Mairangi Bay, Auckland 10, NZ
Phone: 64-9478-592   Fax: 4-9478-5991
Penguin Books
Phone: 64-9415-4700   Fax: 64-9415-4701

UNITED KINGDOM

The Nutri Centre,
Hale Clinic 7 Park Cres, London WIN 3HE
Phone: 44-171-436-5122   Fax: 4-171-636-0276
The Grove - Holistic Medical Clinic
182-184 Kensington Church St. W8 4DP
Phone: 44-171-221-2266   Fax: 44-171-243-2112
Deep Books
Unit13 Cannon Wharf Business Centre, 35 Evelyn St. London SE85 RT
Phone: 44-171-232-2747   Fax: 44-171-237-0067

W.H.A.S. Books & Publications

These books written by Dr. Sandra Cabot are available from most book stores and health food outlets, or can be obtained by using the International Contact Information on page 294, of this book.

THE LIVER CLEANSING DIET BOOK
- 8 week detox diet plan
- 12 vital principles

THE BODY SHAPING DIET BOOK
- Understand the 4 Body Types
- Learn how to shape up
- Maintain your correct Body Type
- Vital links between hormonal balance and weight

BOOST YOUR ENERGY BOOK
- Understand the immune system
- Learn about the latest hormone technology
- Learn how to increase energy

WOMEN'S HEALTH BOOK
Published by Pan
- Holistic healing approach
- Covers all women's health problems

DON'T LET HORMONES RUIN YOUR LIFE BOOK
- Premenstrual syndrome
- Postnatal depression
- Unwanted facial hair, acne and poor libido etc
- Headaches

THE HANDBAG HEALTH GUIDE BOOK
- Quick reference guide, a tiny book to keep handy
- Common health problems
- Natural easy solutions

MENOPAUSE-HRT & IT'S NATURAL ALTERNATIVES BOOK
- Anti-aging plan
- Natural HRT
- Phytoestrogens

BROCHURES ON NATURAL HEALTH PRODUCTS AVAILABLE FREE OF CHARGE
- Latest up to date information
- Contact W.H.A.S. Australia

It is the policy of SCB International Inc. and W.H.A.S. to promote and support its International distributors. However, if you have difficulty obtaining any of the books or brochures mentioned above, please contact the American or Australian office, details on page 294, for mail order.

Glossary- Recipes

Arrowroot - Is similar to cornstarch and is also used as a thickening agent. It can be used to thicken soups and gravies, instead of flour, and in baking biscuits and cakes. Is gluten free.

Banana Leaf - Young banana leaves can be used for cooking and wrapping food. They can be bought and trimmed to size. Always cut the mid rib away. Most Asian shops and grocers will stock them. I have even seen them in some supermarkets. They will keep in the freezer for several months.

Carob Flour - Made from the carob bean, may be a substitute whenever chocolate or cocoa is used.

Coconut - When buying dessicated or shredded coconut always sniff the packet, it will smell rancid if it is off, even through the plastic.

Coconut Milk - Is the white milky liquid that is extracted from the flesh with hot water, not the milk inside the coconut. It can be bought from the supermarket or Asian stores.

Cold Pressed Oil - All oils i.e., olive, almond, walnut, canola, avocado, flaxseed, etc. should be stored in the dark, either under the sink or in a cupboard as this extends the shelf life and stops them from going rancid. If buying oil in large quantities, store the main container and use a funnel to pour the oil into a dark or green glass bottle for daily use.

Couscous - Is made from semolina (not gluten free) and can be used in sweet and savoury dishes. Is an alternative to rice and pasta.

Dry Roast - To place either nuts, seeds, spices and some flours in a heavy saucepan, without any liquid, and constantly moved over a high flame to release the flavour, aroma and natural oils. A delicious seasoning.

Filo Pastry - A very thin pastry made from flour and water. It can be bought frozen or freshly made. When using filo keep it covered as it tends to dry out.

Fish Sauce - A dark coloured sauce used mainly in Asian cooking. It is made from anchovies marinated in vinegar and water.

Flour - There are many types of flour, that can be used for cooking. Mung bean, carob, chestnut, oat, buckwheat, barley, rice (brown, white, black and red rice), arrowroot, amaranth, quinoa, spelt, chickpea (Besan), corn, rye, soy, lentil, potato and wheat to name a few. To make the flour self raising add 1 teaspoon of BAKING POWDER.

Some ideas of whole wheat substitution might be

1 cup of whole wheat flour (plain) $=$ 1/2 cup soy $+$ 1/2 cup arrowroot

or any one of the following

3/4 cup rice flour
1 cup corn flour
1 $+$ 1/4 cups barley flour
3/4 cup potato flour
1 $+$ 1/3 cups oat flour
1 $+$ 1/3 cups soy flour

Julienne - The name given to food strips, (firm foods are easier to work with), ie. carrots, chillis, ginger, celery etc, cut into thin, long strips.

Marinate - To soak foods in a liquid mixture, to either flavour, soften (tenderise) or preserve.

Miso - A paste made from fermented beans, usually soya. Other varieties include, barley and rice. Sweet or savoury. It can be used to make a quick nutritious soup, stock, or spread on bread.

Mushrooms - There are many delicious varieties, shiitake, field (wild), porcini and button to name a few. When exploring Asian green grocers and shops, keep an eye out for exotic and delicious fresh and dried varieties. Experiment with a combination of mushrooms for the various recipes. When using dried mushrooms, always soak in water for approximately 30 minutes before cooking. Are a source of selenium and are good for the immune system.

Palm Sugar - A reddish brown sugar, can be grated or dissolved and used in any recipe instead of sugar.

Purée - To make foods into a smooth consistancy using a blender, food processor or masher.

Rice Noodles - Made from rice and water. Available in different thicknesses, from a flat wide noodle to thin vermicelli. The thin variety can be soaked in hot water for 20 minutes. Can be bought fresh or dried.

Sambal - A hot and spicy relish, usually made from crushed chillies and vinegar.

Seaweeds - are really sea vegetables. They are very high in trace minerals and calcium, and are good for the bones and immune system. Can be used in soups, stirfries and other dishes. Some tasty varities are, Hijiki, Nori, Kombu, Agar Agar, Arame and Wakame.

> **Agar Agar** - Is made from sea vegetables and used to set jellies and mousses etc. It can be used exactly like gelatin. It needs to be cooked or simmered for several minutes in water before setting.
>
> **Arame** - A thin (thread), black sea vegetable. Great in salads and rice.
>
> **Hijiki** - A nutty, salty sea vegetable. Before adding to soups and stirfries, soak for around 10 minutes.
>
> **Kombu** - Is a large, flat, dark green sea vegetable. It is mainly used for stocks and soups. Good with beans and other vegetables.
>
> **Nori** - Comes in dark brown or green sheets or ribbons. It is a sea vegetable and is generally used to make sushi. It can be bought toasted or plain, when using nori to make sushi, it needs to be toasted slightly.
>
> To toast - quickly pass over a gas flame on each side, till crispy. Store in an airtight container in a dark place.
>
> **Wakame** - A long, thin sea vegetable. Good for stocks and soups. It can be used dry, if baked - crumbled on top of salads and vegetable dishes.

Shoyu - is very similar to soy, but is not chemically processed. It is a little sweeter and slightly more salty than tamari.

Soy Sauce - Available as either dark (a little sweeter) or light (saltier), and is made from fermented soya beans and wheat. Look for naturally brewed soy sauces that do not contain chemical additives.

Tamari - is similar to soy and shoyu but is less salty and has no wheat. Is very tasty and can be used whenever soy sauce is needed, as a wheat/gluten free substitute. Is a by product of the miso making process.

Tempeh - is made mainly from fermented soybeans, but can be made from other beans and nuts. It has a very nutty flavour and is more firm and compact than tofu. Can be used interchangeably with tofu.

Tahini - Is a paste made from toasted/untoasted sesame seeds. It can be either hulled(white) or unhulled (brownish). It is very high in calcium and good for the bones. Great for spreads, dressings, sauces etc.

Tofu - Is made from soybeans. It is low in calories and fat, and is cholesterol free. Great for those who are wanting to loose weight, it can be used in soups, desserts and stirfry dishes. Can be substituted for most chicken and many of the seafood dishes in this book.

Umeboshi - A pickled plum which has a salty/ sour taste. It is used for salad dressings, with vegetables and is great with rice.

Wok - Basically it is an Asian saucepan. It has sloping sides and is very handy. When the ingredients at the bottom are cooked, they can be moved up the side and the uncooked ingredients moved down. It can be used to steam, stirfry and also deep fry any foods.

Glossary- Medical

Amino Acids- a group of organic compounds identified by the presence of both an amino group (NH2) and a carboxyl group (COOH). They are the building blocks for protein and are essential to life. Although around 80 amino acids are found in nature, only 22 are needed for human metabolism. The ones that cannot be produced by the body, and must be supplied by food, are called essential amino acids. The essential amino acids are histidine, isoleucine, leucine, lysine, methionine, cysteine, phenylalanine, tyrosine, threonine, tryptophan, and valine. The non-essential amino acids (which the body can manufacture itself), are alanine, aspartic acid, arginine, citrulline, glutamic acid, glycine, hydroxyglutamic acid, hydroxyproline, norleucine, proline and serine. Arginine can be essential in certain states or age groups because the body cannot make it fast enough to supply the demand.

Anus - the outlet of the rectum through which faeces are expelled. It is found between the buttocks.

Autoantibodies - proteins formed by the immune system (known as immunoglobulins), which attack the tissues of the body in which they are formed.

Autoimmune Disease - diseases where the immune system is unable to distinguish its own tissues from foreign substances. The immune system produces antibodies against normal body tissues, which results in inflammation and injury.

Bacteria - microorganisms that can be shaped as a sphere, a rod or a spiral. They grow in colonies, usually composed of the descendants of a single cell. All animals and humans carry bacteria on and in their bodies, and some have the potential to cause serious diseases. Many bacteria produce toxins. Bacteria are the principle agents of decay and putrefaction of organic substances.

Carcinogenic - capable of causing cancer.

Cat Scan (CAT) - computerised X Ray, looking at the body in slices.

Chlorophyll - the green pigment found in plants, which absorbs sunlight. This pigment has health benefits when consumed.

Chronic - long drawn out illness, with slow progression, opposite of acute.

Cirrhosis- a chronic disease of the liver characterized by formation of scar tissue in the liver and destruction of normal liver cells.

Colonic Irrigation - washing or flushing out the colon with enemas, consisting of large amounts of fluid.

Colitis - inflammation of the colon

Cryotherapy - the freezing of abnormal and/or unwanted tissue to destroy it.

Damaged Fats - dietary fats whose chemical structure has been changed from its natural state by oxidation induced by light, heat and oxygen or chemical manufacturing processes.

Dairy Products - animal milks and their products such as butter, cheese, cream, yoghurt, icecream and chocolate.

Detoxification - reduction of the toxic properties of a poisonous substance.

Digestion - the process of breaking food down into smaller particles, so it can be absorbed into the blood stream and utilized by the body.

Dysfunction - impaired, inadequate or abnormal function of an organ, or part of the body.

Enzymes - complex protein substances produced by living cells. Enzymes act as catalysts and induce chemical changes in other substances without being changed themselves. Enzymes are present in digestive juices, where they act upon food substances, breaking them down into smaller simpler substances. They are present in every cell, especially in the liver and enable the liver cells to breakdown drugs and toxins. They can speed up chemical reactions and processes involved in both breaking down substances or building new substances.

Essential Fatty Acids - the unsaturated fatty acids that cannot be manufactured by the body and are essential to good health. These are linolenic acid, arachidonic acid and linoleic acid, and are obtained in certain foods (see page 20)

Fats - substances made up of one molecule of glycerol combined with three fatty acids. The fats found in body tissues are made up of fatty acids, especially oleic acid, palmitic acid and stearic acid. See also lipids.

Fat-soluble - substances dissolving in fatty tissues/liquids only.

Fibromyalgia - inflammation and pain in the muscles and ligaments. Commonly occurs in neck and shoulders.

Fungi - a species of plant-like organisms that includes yeasts and moulds. Fungi grow as single cells as in yeast, or as multicellular filamentous colonies, as in moulds and mushrooms. Many forms are pathogenic to animals and plants.

Gallbladder - pear shaped sac on under surface of right lobe of liver holding bile from the liver until it is discharged through the cystic duct into the intestines.

Gastroenterologist - a physician with postgraduate training in the diagnosis and treatment of diseases affecting the digestive system.

Genetic - pertaining to the genes (found on the chromosomes) or DNA of the organism or species. Concerned with hereditary characteristics and reproduction.

Genetic Engineering - the alteration, manufacture or repair of genetic material by synthetic means.

Glandular System - the network of glands that manufacture hormones. Also known as the endocrine system.

Gluten - a protein found in many grains, including wheat, rye, barley and oats.

Haemorrhoid - a mass of dilated veins occurring around the anus or rectum.

Hepatitis - inflammation of the liver.

Hepatologist - a physician with special training in the diagnosis and treatment of liver diseases.

Hiatus hernia - a protrusion of a portion of the stomach up through the diaphragm into the chest cavity.

HRT - hormone replacement therapy.

Hormone - a chemical, such as a complex protein or steroid substance produced by the various glands in the body. Hormones act as messenger chemicals and give the cells directions. For example thyroid hormone speeds up metabolism, while oestrogen causes breast tissue to grow. The liver breaks down hormones.

Hydrogenation - a chemical process used to turn liquid oils into solid form. This is achieved by passing hydrogen atoms through the oil under high pressure. Hydrogenation impairs the nutritional value of the oil and produces distorted fatty acid molecules that do not occur in nature.

Hypoglycaemia - abnormally low level of sugar (glucose) in the blood.

Immune System - a system that exists in the body to identify and eliminate foreign and harmful substances or microorganisms that have invaded the body. It consists of specialized cells that produce antibodies and/or ingest these foreign things. The lymphatic system, bone marrow, thymus gland, spleen and liver, all play vital roles in the efficient functioning of the immune system.

Immunoglobulins - proteins manufactured by the cells of the immune system that attack or neutralize foreign substances or microorganisms. They are also known as antibodies.

Infection - invasion of body tissues by disease causing microorganisms, such as viruses, protozoa, bacteria or fungi.

Inflammation - redness, heat, swelling, disintegration and sometimes pain, occurring in tissues injured by various means such as infection, burning, excess acidity, trauma or toxins.

Jaundice - yellow discolouration of the skin and mucous membranes caused by a build up in the body of bile pigments.

Kupffer Cells - specialized cells inside the sinusoids of the liver, which remove and destroy toxic rubbish from the blood in the sinusoidal spaces. They are known as phagocyte cells because they ingest and destroy rubbish. These cells are vitally important to healthy liver function.

Lactase - an enzyme that exists in the intestinal lining and is required to digest the sugar found in milk (lactose).

Lactose Intolerance - an inability of the body to metabolize the sugar found in milk (lactose) which is due to deficiency of the enzyme lactase. Symptoms include diarrhoea, abdominal cramps, bloating and gas.

Lipase - the enzyme produced by the pancreas that breaks down fats into smaller absorbable substances.

Lipids - fatty substances which are insoluble in water, and dissolve in fat solvents such as chloroform and alcohol. Lipids include esters of fatty acids and glycerol, phospholipids and cholesterol.

Lipoma - fatty tumour underneath the skin.

Lipoproteins - molecules consisting of proteins combined with lipids such as cholesterol, phospholipids and triglycerides. Blood fats do not circulate in an unbound or free state, but are chemically bound to proteins, which enables them to be transported safely.

Lymphocytes - white blood cells forming part of the immune system.

Mad Cow Disease - A severe degenerative disease effecting the nervous system in cattle. Transmitted by tiny particles, called prions, found in some forms of stock feed and some animal by-products.

Malnutrition - deficiency of nutrients essential to health

Metastases - deposits of cancer cells that are growing in sites of the body distant to their source of origin.

Microorganisms - minute living bodies, not perceived by the naked eye, eg. a bacterium or parasite. Can be carried from one host to another.

Metabolism - the physical and energy transformations that exist within living cells.

Mitochondria - the energy factories inside every cell.

Mucous - the viscous (glue-like) secretions of the mucous membranes composed of mucin, salts and body cells.

Oesophagus - that portion of the digestive tract that extends from the back of the throat to the stomach. On average it measures 10 to 12 inches in the adult.

Oleuropein - active principle extracted from olive leaves. Has antibiotic properties.

Oxidation - the chemical process in which oxygen reacts with another substance, causing it to change. These changes usually result in some damage or deterioration (similar to rust). Oxidation often liberates free radicals, which cause further damage.

Pancreas - a gland situated behind the stomach. It lies in a horizontal position with its head attached to the duodenum and its tail reaching to the spleen. It produces digestive enzymes which enter the duodenum, and the hormones insulin and glucagon which control glucose metabolism.

Pancreatitis - inflammation of the pancreas.

Parasite - an organism that lives within, upon, or at the expense of another organism, known as the host, without contributing to survival of the host.

Pathogenic - capable of producing disease.

Pernicious Anaemia - severe form of blood anaemia, caused by the deficiency of vitamin B12.

Petrochemical - any chemical obtained from petroleum.

Petroleum - mineral oil found in upper strata of earth and used for fuels and in the manufacture of different chemicals such as many plastics.

Phytonutrients - nutritional substances beneficial to health found in plants.

Protease - an enzyme produced by the pancreas to breakdown food proteins into smaller amino acids.

Pruritus - chronically itchy skin.

Sinusoidal system - the spaces in-between the liver cells which filter toxins and microorganisms out of the blood stream. The sinusoids act like a filter.

Thyroid Gland - small gland, situated in front of the neck, which produces thyroid hormone.

Tumour - swelling or enlargement. A spontaneous new growth of tissue, forming an abnormal mass.

Villi - the finger like projections covering the surface of the inner lining of the intestines that are designed to increase the absorptive area of the intestinal tract.

Virus - a minute organism not visible with ordinary light microscopy. It is a parasite dependent upon nutrients inside cells for its metabolic and reproductive needs. Viruses can be seen by using an electron microscope and consist of a strand of either DNA or RNA (but not both) surrounded by a protein covering.

Water-soluble - substances dissolving in watery tissues/liquids only.

The Liver Tonics Designed for Today's World

We live in a world where we are exposed to polluted air and water, rapidly spreading liver viruses, and foods contaminated with growth promoting hormones, antibiotics, processed fats, insecticides, pesticides, petrochemicals and artificial colourings and sweeteners. This sounds terrible but has become fact - when you sit down to your next meal think about how many toxic chemicals are entering your body. This is not what Mother Nature intended for human beings and we are paying the price with a much higher incidence of cancer and degenerative diseases.

To deal with all these chemicals, the liver is working harder than ever before in the history of mankind. Little wonder that our livers cannot always cope and are often overloaded, toxic and fatty. For these reasons Dr. Sandra Cabot. M.D. has formulated the Livatone range of products to support your liver function and reduce liver damage.

LIVATONE

Contains the liver herbs Milk Thistle, Globe Artichoke and Dandelion combined with Taurine, Lecithin, Pectin, psyllium husks, slippery elm, alfalfa powder, barley leaf powder, Peppermint leaf and carrot and beetroot powder.

ACTIONS:
- Improves liver and gall bladder function
- Cleanses the bowel
- Increases dietary fibre

LIVATONE PLUS

Contains the liver herb Milk Thistle combined with the liver amino acids Taurine, Cysteine, Glutamine and Glycine, powerful antioxidants (Vitamins C & E & carotenoids), the B group vitamins and other vital lipotrophic factors.

ACTIONS:
- Improves the fat burning action of the liver, which aids weight loss
- Reduces fatty liver and fat build up in other organs
- Improves liver and gall bladder function
- Improves the ability of the liver to break down toxic chemicals and drugs
- Detoxifies the liver
- Improves ability of the liver to detoxify alcohol
- Improves liver function in those with liver disease
- Reduces liver damage in those exposed to liver viruses and/or toxins
- Increases liver glutathione

Livatone and Livatone Plus are available in capsule or powder form and are all natural dietary supplements that are safe to take on a long term basis. They do not interact with any prescription drugs or hormones. Directions for their use are found on the label.

Other Products Formulated By DR. SANDRA CABOT

SELENOMUNE POWDER

This powder is made from Brewer's yeast enriched with trace minerals, antioxidants, kelp and vegetable powders. It is high in the powerful antioxidant mineral Selenium and also contains boron, magnesium, chromium and molybdenum.

ACTIONS:
- Improves function of the thyroid gland
- Increases metabolism
- Aids weight loss
- Boosts cellular energy production
- Exerts an anti-viral effect (reduces viral replication)
- Strengthens the immune system
- Reduces inflammation — this effect is beneficial to those with auto immune disease

It is an all natural dietary supplement that is safe to take on a long term basis.

FemmePhase - The Superfood for Your Hormones

FemmePhase is a combination of the herbs (black cohosh, dong quai, wild yam, sage, liquorice, kelp and horsetail) and the foods (alfalfa, soyabean protein and flaxseed) that are high in plant hormones. These plant hormones are called phytoestrogens and exert a balancing effect on your body's hormones. In FemmePhase these herbs and foods are combined with four different types of calcium plus magnesium, zinc, B group vitamins and a full range of natural antioxidant vitamins. It is hard to believe that so many different health promoting ingredients can be found in just one product - that's why FemmePhase is called a superfood!

ACTIONS:
- Reduces symptoms of menopause
- Reduces premenstrual syndrome
- Increases bone density and reduces osteoporosis
- Strengthens nails
- Thickens the hair (take with Selenomune for extra benefit on the hair)
- Improves general well being

Available in capsule or powder form.

FLAXSEED PLUS Capsules

This product combines **cold pressed** Flaxseed oil with Primrose oil and Lecithin. It provides an optimal balance of the omega 3 & 6 essential fatty acids and will improve the cell membranes, which will make your cells more resistant to disease.

ACTIONS:
- Improves brain function and memory
- Reduces the risk of dementia in later life
- Improves mood and sleep
- Improves skin and hair
- Strengthens the immune system.

METABOCEL - Natural Weight Loss Tablets

Are you tired of all those weight loss drugs that have side effects and damage your metabolism permanently? Dr Cabot's all natural METABOCEL, contains super-strength Brindleberry herb which has been proven in clinical trials to prevent fat deposits forming in your body. METABOCEL combines 5500mg of Brindleberry with other natural synergistic ingredients to help the fat burning factories inside every cell of your body. It also enhances thyroid function, which stimulates metabolism. Remember - you will never stay slim unless your metabolism is efficient and that is where METABOCEL can help you- it has been designed to boost metabolism efficiently, safely and naturally. Use METABOCEL in conjunction with the principles of the Liver Cleansing Diet.

To purchase any of these products:

Refer to W.H.A.S. Directory - International Contact Details on page 294 of this book.

If you have any queries or problems Email Dr. Sandra Cabot M.D., the " doctor who understands" at E-mail address:

cabot@ozemail.com.au

Notes

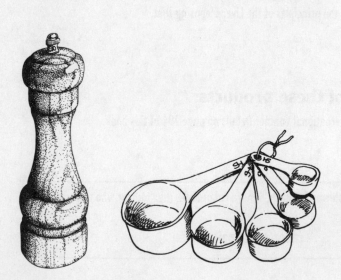